The Ultimate
Introduction to
NLP

The Ultimate
Introduction to

NLP

How to build a
successful life

CO-CREATOR OF NLP

RICHARD BANDLER

ALESSIO ROBERTI & OWEN FITZPATRICK

Thorsons

Thorsons
An imprint of HarperCollins*Publishers*
1 London Bridge Street
London SE1 9GF

www.harpercollins.co.uk

HarperCollins*Publishers*
1st Floor, Watermarque Building, Ringsend Road
Dublin 4, Ireland

First published in 2012 by HarperCollins*Publishers*
This edition published by Thorsons 2017

8

Text © Richard Bandler, Alessio Roberti, Owen Fitzpatrick 2013

The authors assert their moral right to be
identified as the authors of this work

A catalogue record for this book is
available from the British Library

All characters in this book described as attending the NLP
class are fictional. Any resemblance to real persons, living
or dead, is purely coincidental.

ISBN: 978-0-00-749741-6

Printed and bound by CPI Group (UK) Ltd, Croydon, CR0 4YY

MIX
Paper from
responsible sources
FSC™ C007454

This book is produced from independently certified FSC™ paper
to ensure responsible forest management.

For more information visit: www.harpercollins.co.uk/green

CONTENTS

ACKNOWLEDGEMENTS

This book would have never seen the light of day were it not for amazing help from the following people. We send out a huge thank you to all of them for their support, suggestions and hard work in making this book possible.

First to our agent, Robert Kirby, for his phenomenal support, hard work and belief in this book. Robert is a true professional, and his patience, insights and advice proved incredibly valuable.

Thanks to the wonderful team at HarperCollins, especially Carole Tonkinson and Victoria McGeown, who have been superb in their support and their faith in the book.

And last but not least, we thank all of our colleagues, the seminar attendees, support staff and Society of NLP trainers all over the world. Without you, there would be no life-changing seminars.

From Richard

I would like to thank my wife, Glenda, for her help, support and magical smile.

My thanks also go to 40 years of clients who faced the worst and taught me so much.

Thanks also to John and Kathleen La Valle for their friendship and ongoing assistance and encouragement.

From Alessio

I would like to thank Dr Richard Bandler, whose creativity and generosity in sharing his fabulous discoveries have made a significant contribution to my life and the entire field of personal change.

I owe an incredible debt of gratitude to John and Kathleen La Valle, who have supported, encouraged and championed my work so far. Their continuing feedback has helped me develop my NLP and coaching skills.

Thanks to the co-director of the NLP Italy Coaching School, Antonella Rizzuto, whose dedication helps more than 10,000 people every year to discover their potential.

And thanks to Mattia Bernardini and Alice Rifelli, whose professional and diligent work makes life-changing books possible.

Finally, I would like to thank the two most extraordinary people in my life, Cinzia and Damiamo, my world of love.

ACKNOWLEDGEMENTS

From Owen

I would like to thank my parents, Marjorie and Brian Fitzpatrick – quite simply the greatest parents one could wish to have and the people I look up to most in life.

Thanks to my gorgeous goddaughters, Lucy and Aoife, whose beauty makes me smile every day.

And to my incredible friends, including Brian, Theresa, Cristina, Sandra, Gillian, Elena, Kate and Rob, for their advice and support with the book.

My thanks also go to all my trainers and mentors over the years, particularly John and Kathleen La Valle for their invaluable advice. They have, quite simply, changed my life.

Lastly, thank you to Dr Richard Bandler. Meeting Richard as a teenager, I found his genius, advice and belief in me literally turned my world around. I'm blessed to have him as a teacher, mentor and friend in my life.

INTRODUCTION

A workshop between two covers, this is Richard Bandler's most accessible book to date. It's the story of a man named Joe who attends a one-day introductory course on NLP with Dr Richard Bandler, listens to Richard teaching, practises the techniques he teaches, meets other participants and learns as they all share their thoughts and insights on how to apply the content of the course in different areas of their personal and professional lives.

By reading this book, you too can become one of the participants of the course, hearing what they hear, seeing what they see, experiencing what they experience and learning what they learn!

We decided to write a story in which the participants of a course were the protagonists because it's the participants who are at the centre of our training, each with their own needs, ambitions, problems, and desires, each looking for new ideas, tools and solutions.

For many years we were ourselves participants on Richard's courses. We then both became trainers, working as assistants on Richard's international courses for more than a decade. Nowadays, we are lucky to have become international trainers, sharing what we have learned from Richard all over the world. So, it's a great pleasure and honour for us to co-author this book with him and share what we've learned from him and our students so far.

We have written this book because we believe there is a huge need for the core message of these pages to be shared globally. The world is changing rapidly and bringing with it the paradoxical realization that we have been given more and more resources than ever before and modern technology has allowed us to do amazing and wonderful things, yet depression, anxiety, fear, panic and stress are all still on the rise.

The core message of this book is that there are precise tools that can help you to take control of your life. In it, Richard is going to teach you how you can change your thinking and change your life – and how you can help others change their lives too.

We began writing this book in Rome, continued it in Dublin, worked on it in London and New York, and got feedback from people in Los Angeles, Tokyo and even Australia. It is the result of 20 years of interviewing thousands of people who have attended NLP workshops, the product of participants who shared their own experiences with us. It is an international project focused not on NLP but on how people can learn to use NLP to change their lives.

There is a huge need in the world today for a change in mentality. There is a huge need to inject hope for a better world. We stand at an important crossroads between letting ourselves be pushed along by the accelerating momentum of challenging circumstances or deciding to steer ourselves to where we want to go. We need a change of direction. We need a change of consciousness. We need to know that we can have a say in how the world turns out.

NLP is a movement. You can be part of it. Start now – it's your time!

Alessio and Owen

Chapter 1

A WORKSHOP WITH THE CO-CREATOR OF NLP

Joe put his phone back into his pocket, took a deep breath and composed himself. Having just had an argument with his girl-friend, he certainly wasn't in the best of moods. That said, he knew it was really important to get the most out of the day. He walked into the lobby of the hotel, where he immediately noticed a familiar face among the assistants taking care of registration.

Joe smiled. Seeing Alan cheered him up a bit.

'Joe!' Alan called out. 'Fantastic to see you again.'

'Likewise,' Joe replied. 'Yeah, I've been really looking forward to today. Finally I decided to find out more about this NLP stuff.'

NLP stood for 'Neuro-Linguistic Programming'. Having seen many books on the topic, Joe had a sense of how popular it was. He'd understood it was an attitude and methodology that allowed people to think and communicate more effectively, and he needed to do both. Up until a year before, he had resigned himself to the idea that he was the way he was and his life was what it was and there was nothing he could do about it. But then he had learned that things could change, and now he really wanted to work on himself and make some improvements.

'Just to give you the heads up on what's in store,' Alan began, 'you've already seen Richard in action. Today, you'll learn about the field of NLP itself.'

Alan was referring to Dr Richard Bandler, the co-founder of NLP. Joe had met Richard at a course he had attended a year previously. At the time, he had been alone and depressed. To help out, his sister, Maria, had given him a flyer for a three-day course entitled 'Choose Freedom', which had involved a workshop with Dr Bandler. That was where he had met Alan, who had been an assistant at the course.

Now Alan was saying, 'And as ever, I'll be around to help in any way I can.'

'Great,' Joe replied. 'It's much appreciated.'

Over the three days of the previous course, Joe had gradually come to the realization that it was possible to change things even when challenges seemed insurmountable. Now he was keen to learn more.

'So, what are the highlights of today?'

'Well, you'll learn some remarkable strategies for accessing powerful emotional states, getting better at communicating with others and really improving the different areas of your life.

Probably the best way to describe this stuff is that it's the difference that makes the difference. It's how to build a successful life.'

Joe really needed to succeed at this moment in time. He was facing two important issues. You see, after the first course, things had really changed for him. He had a good job now and a good relationship with a girl he was crazy about. He had everything he could wish for. But that meant he had a lot to lose. In fact he was feeling more nervous now than he had 12 months before! When he hadn't really had much of a life, it hadn't mattered much what happened to him or what he did. But now he knew that he needed to do something, and soon, if he wanted to hold on to the things that mattered to him.

Alan took him to one side. 'So, how's everything going? How's that beautiful girlfriend of yours?'

'She's fine. I mean, we were getting on great … but nothing's perfect, I suppose. It's just that now – well, we're considering moving in together.'

'Moving in together? Wow! That's fantastic news, Joe. I expect an invite to the big day!'

'Hold your horses, Alan. Marriage is a whole other story! It is great, though.'

Joe paused. He knew he wasn't sounding convincing.

'Obviously, we're getting to know each other a lot more now … and we have our differences. So that's taking some getting used to.'

Joe looked down, thinking about the argument he'd just had with his girlfriend.

'Joe,' Alan said seriously, 'if you feel she's the one, you need to make sure you hold on to her. You'll regret it for the rest of your life if you don't.'

As Joe looked up, he noticed a certain intensity in Alan's eyes. What was all that about? He knew Alan was right, but even talking about his relationship made him feel worse. He decided to change the subject.

'Work is a lot better,' he said confidently. 'I got a promotion, so I'm obviously delighted with that. Although,' he went on more slowly, 'I have found myself struggling with the new role at times. I have a lot more interaction with customers now and it's just … I don't think I'm a very good people person.'

Suddenly aware that Alan was studying him, he felt embarrassed.

'Anyway, I make it sound worse than it actually is. I just think there are a few things NLP could help me with. You asked!'

He smiled sheepishly.

'Just remember,' Alan said, smiling back, 'there's no such thing as a *people person*. What can help is to learn to feel comfortable around others and become better at communicating with them.'

Joe nodded.

'The seminar should help,' Alan said reassuringly. 'That's it, you're registered now, Joe. Best of luck!'

'Thanks!'

No sooner had Joe turned around and started to walk towards the seminar room than he saw another familiar face.

Teresa, an Irish doctor he had met at his first seminar with Richard Bandler, threw her arms around him.

'Joe, what a lovely surprise! Allow me to introduce my beautiful daughter, Emily.'

Emily looked to be in her mid to late teens. She had long red hair and was dressed in jeans and a Minnie Mouse t-shirt. She smiled politely as she shook hands with Joe.

'So,' Joe said, hoping to break the ice, 'are you also new to all this, or am I the only one?'

'I'm a first-timer,' Emily replied. 'I've just read a couple of books we have at home, that's all. *She's* the NLP expert of the family.' She gestured towards her mother with her thumb. 'You know what they say: "An old broom knows the dirty corners best."'

'Very funny, dear, but the only dirty corners I know are in your room!' Teresa said in her warm, maternal voice. 'Sure, I've been studying NLP for a couple of years, and I use it in my daily practice as well as in my personal life, but I'm no expert. In fact, the best lesson I learned from NLP is that "you're never done learning", as they say, so if you have the feeling that you know everything there is to know, you're obviously missing out on something! And the worst thing is that you're so blinded by your own certainty that you don't even realize that you're missing it.'

'Wow,' Joe said to Emily with a cheeky smile, 'your mum's cool!'

'The best,' Emily confirmed. 'Sometimes I wonder if she's for real!'

'Oh, come on, you two!' And with that, Teresa playfully slapped Joe's shoulder.

As the three of them made their way towards the seminar room, Joe and Teresa began to catch up on what had been happening since they had last met. At one point, they stopped talking for a moment as they noticed a lady rummaging through her handbag. She was red-faced and looked extremely worried. Then, just as Joe and Teresa were about to ask if she was OK, she heaved a deep sigh of relief as she pulled a small mirror out of her bag.

Joe and Teresa exchanged glances, and he shook his head. *All that stress over a makeup mirror*, he thought. *If this seminar is anything like the last, she's really going to benefit from it.*

Joe, Teresa and Emily went into the seminar room and found three seats together halfway up the centre aisle. Joe found himself placed between Teresa and a man in his fifties wearing a sharp suit and a pair of red designer glasses.

'Hi, I'm Joe.'

'Edgar Martin's the name, changing lives is the game,' said the man with a laugh. 'Nice to meet you, Joe. What brings you here today?'

Joe grinned. 'Long story short? A year ago I was in a bad place in my life and struggling with things. My sister convinced me to go to a seminar and, well, that turned some things around for me. I know NLP was involved, so I'm here to learn about it. How about you?'

'That's an interesting path you took, Joe,' Edgar said. 'I'm here to add a few tools to my toolbox, so to speak. I'm not a plumber, though. Well, maybe a plumber of the mind!' Once again he laughed at his own joke. 'I'm a psychiatrist and a psychotherapist.'

Joe smiled politely. 'Cool,' he said as he took out his personal journal.

'Nice journal there, Joe,' Edgar commented. 'Do you take it everywhere you go?'

Joe nodded. 'Well, not *everywhere*.' He winked as he tried to match Edgar's sense of humour, but all he got was a blank stare in response. Slightly red-faced, he continued, 'I know from the last time that Richard Bandler teaches through stories, so you absorb a lot of ideas unconsciously, yet I also wanted to consciously capture some of his most memorable insights and observations throughout the workshop. I find taking notes to be a great way to review the key concepts and techniques.'

Edgar looked impressed. 'It didn't occur to me to bring along a journal, but I might look for one at the first break. Although really I should have brought my iPad – so I could have synchronized my database up here with my external memory!'

Pointing to his head, Edgar laughed again, while Joe nodded, this time failing to smile.

'This is my first time learning from Richard,' Edgar continued. 'It's just ... I got so much from Alan, my first NLP trainer, that I figured it was time I learned from his mentor. Actually, Alan's here today too, as an assistant.'

'Oh, yes, I know Alan,' Joe replied, suddenly intrigued. 'What's he like as a trainer?'

Before Edgar could answer, music began and Richard Bandler appeared at the back of the room. With a glance and a nod of the head, Edgar and Joe silently agreed to postpone their conversation. The seminar was about to begin.

Chapter 2

A BRIEF HISTORY OF NLP

As Richard Bandler walked towards the stage, Joe stared at him curiously. He had heard that top executives, Olympic athletes and even presidents of countries had benefited from NLP, but he still wasn't sure what it was all about. He really wanted to understand it properly, and as Richard Bandler had been one of the co-creators of the field in the early 1970s, this seminar seemed the perfect place to start. He opened his journal as Richard began to speak:

Let me begin by giving you the background to all of this. When it started out – well, it was actually a fluke. My training was primarily in mathematics, logic and science, and when I was in college I moved into a house owned by a psychiatrist, and it was filled with books. Being an avid reader, I started reading them, waiting to get to the point where they said what you could do to help a patient.

Unfortunately the only book that I found that told you how to do anything was the book that told you how to prescribe drugs. If people were depressed, you could prescribe antidepressants for them. The worst part was that many of the people who took antidepressants were still depressed. It's not much good when you take the drug and you go, 'My life is still all screwed up.'

Being the practical guy that I am, I couldn't believe that was it, so I started investigating further.

Now, if there's one thing that's kept me moving over the years, it's the will to find simple ways to do difficult things. And this search has brought me in touch with some truly amazing human beings. Today I'll tell you a little about some of them and the things I had the chance to learn from them.

In the beginning, all I did was go out and explore how people behaved: I was convinced there had to be a better way to organize information about how humans do things. When I met schizophrenics, I thought they were much like my neighbours – I couldn't really tell the difference. They just had different ways of thinking about the world than others did. Their models or maps didn't match other people's experience.

In fact, the concept that the map is not the territory is one of the ideas that laid the foundations of Neuro-Linguistic Programming. It means that your understanding of the world is based on how you represent it – your map – and not on the world itself.

Joe had the feeling that this was important, so he paid close attention as Richard continued:

In order to understand the world, we map it in our brain. make a map, you go through three basic processes.

First, you delete part of the information. On a city m don't draw the cars, you don't see what the rooftops look lik., and so on. And this a useful process – until you delete something important like a whole block of buildings and then try to drive through it because your map says there's nothing there.

How many of you have experienced this: you're walking down a familiar street and all of a sudden you notice what looks like a new shop. You walk in, ask how long it's been open and find out it's been there for five years!

The audience nodded. Joe remembered having that experience often.

Next, when making a map, you generalize. On a map, all state roads are represented the same way, regardless of how they actually look, and when you see a blue-coloured shape you expect it to be a lake or the sea.

Generalization is part of the learning process. You play with fire, you get burned, you learn not to touch things when they're too hot. It's a good thing. But then you have a partner who cheats on you and you decide all men are pigs – that might be an over-generalization. It's not the process itself that is good or bad, it's when and how you use it.

Last, you distort part of the information. A city map is usually smaller than the city itself, right? And it's flat: it's a print on a piece of paper. In life, you distort information every time you blow things out of proportion, whether you make them bigger than they actually are or whether you make them smaller.

Another, subtler way you distort things is this: you attach meaning to something that happened, or something that someone said or did. A colleague enters the room and she doesn't greet you: you figure she's angry, or upset, or offended.

And again, I don't mean to say that distortion is necessarily a bad thing. In fact, it can lead to fairly accurate conclusions. What's important is that you realize there's a process going on and that the way you see things and the way they really are may be very different. And most important of all: whatever you think is going on, I want you to remember that it's just a map. And it doesn't necessarily match the map of the people around you.

Think about that the next time you end up arguing about who's right and who's wrong. As long as you stay with your own map, you'll also stay convinced that you're probably right. And the other person will stay convinced they're probably right. When your map and the maps of the people around you don't match, that's when the trouble begins.

Once I realized that, I understood that in order to have better options, better feelings, better interactions with others, you need to expand your map. You need to be able to look at the same things from different perspectives. The more detailed your map is, the more freedom and flexibility you have.

Joe jotted down in his journal what he was taking from this. He thought about his relationship with his girlfriend, the issues and misunderstandings they had been having recently and how they made him painfully aware of how scared he was of losing her. He loved her, but he would often find himself taking offence to what she said and believing that she didn't understand him and was growing distant from him. Now he realized that she obviously had her map and her way of thinking about their relationship, just as he had his.

As he continued to listen to Richard, Joe decided that it would be a good idea to talk to his girlfriend and find out more about what she was thinking and feeling about things, rather than focusing purely on his own perceptions and concerns.

And Richard was offering valuable guidance:

A good piece of advice is this: do a reality check from time to time. Make sure that your map is up to date, because when people stop looking at what's out there and only rely on their old map, they mess up in one of two ways: either they imagine limits and constraints where there are none, or they act as if something should work, and when it doesn't, they just do more of the same.

I know many of you generalize the experiences you've had so far and then project them into your future. The fact is that your future hasn't been written yet. Life is full of opportunities, and opportunities lie ahead, in the future. Don't let anyone, not even your own map, convince you of the contrary.

For example, just because you have had some negative experiences with your business partners, it doesn't mean that all human beings will stab you in the back over money. Perhaps it means you should learn to protect your interests; perhaps it means that you should change the way you select your business partners.

Imagine what life would be if the future could only be a repetition of what you have already experienced in the past: what a sad, sad world this would be. Not to mention the fact that we would still be living in caves and feeding off raw meat and bitter roots.

Luckily there's an evolutionary drive in the universe, a force so strong that it defies chaos, and that force is what animates human beings.

Joe felt a sense of lightness as he came to a realization. In his journal, he wrote: 'It's not about who's right and who's wrong. It's not about what's "true", either. A good map is a map that gets you to see things from different perspectives and that helps you feel as resourceful as possible about your situation.'

Richard was getting down to what was most important:

Now, NLP isn't something that you can learn just by reading about it or talking about it. You learn NLP through practice! That's why today's programme is rich in techniques and exercises.

I want you to know that even though this is a short workshop, I'm going to put lots of stuff inside your mind that is going to come out later. You might not understand all of it now, but remember, your unconscious is also listening.

This all started with a simple idea: I would go out and find people who had done something successfully, and I would discover the unconscious process that they used.

14

Joe heard Emily whispering to Teresa. 'What does he mean by "unconscious process"?'

Teresa responded quietly, 'Unconscious processes are the recipes that you follow to produce thoughts, feelings and behaviour. By becoming aware of these processes, you can then deliberately improve them or change them.'

Emily nodded as she thought this through.

I would then teach people to consciously engage in these processes, so that their problems would get solved or they could acquire specific skills.

What people *say* they do, or *believe* they do – well, it's often far removed from what they *actually* do.

The thing that, for me, makes NLP revolutionary is this: it's the first time that we have been able to deliberately reshape the inside of our minds. We have the tools to find out where the crap we don't want is and to replace it with things we actually do want.

Joe wasn't convinced. Although his life had changed quite radically since his first seminar experience with Richard, the idea that you could reshape the inside of your mind seemed a bit far-fetched to him.

Richard, however, was moving forward:

You weren't born with your bad habits. You weren't born with your skills. You weren't born with your beliefs. The vast majority of the things that you do, you learned – just like you learned to walk or to shake hands automatically.

Even fears are learned! Do you know there are only two natural fears? The fear of loud noises and the fear of falling – that's it. All the rest are learned. Now, some of them are useful, like being afraid of rattlesnakes, and some of them are less useful. You don't want to get rid of fear altogether; you just want to learn to be afraid of the appropriate thing at the appropriate time. Like having a phobia about cheating on your partner! That's a phobia worth having.

When I started out, people kept telling me things like, 'You don't understand, Richard. Change is slow and painful.'

But I'm not an understanding person – I refuse to accept limiting beliefs just because I'm told to. I believe that most often people change rapidly without any of this nonsense. I mean, all kind of things happen. You watch a movie or read a book, you talk to a friend, or even to a stranger on the bus, and your life is transformed by it. Instantly. You don't need to read the same sentence for 13 years – you just read it once and you go, 'Wow! That makes a lot of sense!'

You can't argue with the man's logic, Joe thought to himself.

And here's another of those things people still tell me: they come to me and go, 'You have to discover who you really are and to accept yourself.' Well, I'm here to tell you you don't. You don't have to be anything you don't want to be. Because you've acted like a shy person up till now doesn't mean you're doomed to play shy for the rest of your life. The fact that you might have acted lazy or

reckless doesn't *make* you so – it's a behavioural pattern
you are. You can be whoever you choose to be.

Change happens all the time – it's the only constant in
point is, are you going to *choose* the direction your life will take
and the kind of person you will become, or will you just sit back
and wait for life to happen to you?

With NLP, you get to change how you think, feel and behave.
You get to take what you are doing – both inside your head and
in the real world – and reprogram yourself so that you can make
powerful changes in your mind. So, you see, here you have the
chance to take control of your life, but it only works if you *do* it
– if you actually commit to doing what it takes to change things
around, and then go and make it happen.

I want to share with you how you can not only feel as good as
you have in the past, but even better than that. It's about being
able to pimp up your brain!

Joe laughed. He loved the idea that you could make changes to
your mind just like that TV show where they took rusty old
wrecks and transformed them into shining supercars! He
remembered how sceptical he had felt when his sister had
suggested that he go on the first seminar. Up to that moment he
had been feeling stuck, out of options, and the idea that he
could choose who he wanted to be – well, that had sounded just
like wishful thinking. Now, he felt different. He listened atten-
tively as Richard continued:

One day, the guy who owned the house I was living in called me and told me that Virginia Satir was going to be staying in the area, so I should keep an eye on her and make sure she was comfortable. Now, Virginia was the reason why I got sidetracked from mathematics and science and ended up co-creating NLP: she was a very talented psychotherapist who could actually produce consistent results.

The first time I saw her, I was outside working on my car, changing an oil filter, and suddenly this woman walked up the driveway. She was a vision: very tall and wearing a Day-Glo green dress, bright red high heels and big horn-rimmed glasses. She was staring at me with a big smile, so I got up, looked at her, and went, 'Can I help you?'

And she said, 'I certainly hope so. I've never used a wood-burning stove and I wouldn't want to set the house on fire.'

As we walked towards her place, I said, 'So, you're Virginia. Everybody says you're a great psychotherapist. What exactly do you do?'

'Well,' she said, 'I don't really do what other people do. I try to get my clients to be happy.'

Now that made a lot of sense to me, so I asked, 'Does it work?'

And she said, 'I've been very fortunate, because I've been able to help many people whom no one else could help.'

'Like who?' I asked.

'Well, I work a lot with schizophrenics who are hospitalized, and I discovered that if you bring their whole family in, some of them don't seem so crazy anymore.'

Being someone who studied systems, I found this very interesting.

So, Virginia offered to take me with her. She was doing some training with the staff in a mental hospital and when I watched her work, everything she did seemed to make perfect sense to me. The questions that she asked were very effective and very systematic, but all I could hear from the staff were things like 'Oh, she's a miracle worker! Isn't she so intuitive?' Translation into human: 'It's not my responsibility to learn these skills, because they're based on who she is, not what she does.'

Virginia understood that the map wasn't the territory and she took that concept to a level that, to me, was a revelation. Of course, she did a whole lot of things – some of which you'll get to learn later today – but basically what she did was, instead of interpreting what people said in a metaphorical sense, she took it literally. When someone told her things didn't 'look' good, she assumed they were talking about a picture inside their head. And if they said something about the 'sound' of things, she knew they were referring to an internal sound. Most importantly, she understood that people needed someone who could 'speak their language', 'see things their way' or, if you prefer, 'grasp their inner world'.

Joe was confused. *What did Richard mean by this?*

Now, let me give you an example that will make things clearer to you. One day Virginia is working with a couple because they are fighting so much their marriage is nearly wrecked.

'He never does anything at home,' the wife begins. 'It *looks* as if he doesn't even live there. I run around all day trying to make the place *look* decent and he just makes a mess out of it.'

And Virginia goes, 'I *see* what you mean, Lucy.'

Guys, this woman keeps describing her pictures, and Virginia acknowledges this.

Then Virginia looks at the husband and goes, 'How about you, Bob?'

Bob says, 'She just *screams* all the time. It's impossible to have a *conversation* with her. One minute everything's *quiet*, then the next thing I know, she's *wailing* about something I don't even know about.'

The husband tends to use lots of auditory or sound words. Do you *hear* that?

Good. So Virginia goes, 'I *hear* you, Bob. Now, Lucy, have you tried *telling* him these things without getting angry first?'

'It's impossible,' Lucy says. '*Look*, I put the trash next to the door so that he *sees* it when he goes out. Will he take it out? No. Then I wait to *see* if he'll take it out when he comes back. In the morning it's still there. Then I see to it myself and when he *shows* up, I'm already fuming.'

'OK,' says Virginia, 'let me *see* if I can give him a clearer *picture*. Bob, you *heard* your wife out. What's your story?'

'It's like I *told* you, like she's *tuned* me out or something. How am I supposed to know what's going on if she doesn't *talk* to me? It's not that I enjoy the regular *screaming and shouting*.'

After a brief negotiation, always matching her words to those of the person she's addressing, Virginia gets Lucy to agree to try *telling* Bob what he's supposed to *see*. In exchange, Lucy gets her way on another hot issue.

'He *tells* me he loves me all the time', Lucy goes, 'but he never *shows* it to me.'

'How would you want him to *show* it to you?' Virginia enquires.

'I'd want him to notice if I put on some nice clothes or did my hair. I'd love it if he came home with flowers.'

'I *see*', says Virginia. 'Let me *show* you something, but you need to *picture* the words as well.'

This is Virginia's way of overlapping Lucy's visual experience with her ability to talk and listen. This is what made her the genius she was.

Then she turns to Bob and translates Lucy's experience into something that he can understand: 'Now, you *listen* to me. Are you aware that when your wife puts on a new dress and you don't *look* at her, it's as if you *told* her in the sweetest *voice* how much you loved her and she turned a *deaf ear* to you?'

'Well', Bob retorts, 'that's exactly what she does.'

'That's because she needs you to *tell* her that you *see* her, that you *watch* her, that you pay attention to how she *looks*. Do you *hear* me on this?'

'*Loud and clear.*' Then to his wife: 'It's when I *look* at you and *see* how beautiful you are that I feel like *telling* you how much I love you. I just didn't realize that needed to be *said out loud*. I'm sorry.'

A smile crossed Joe's face. His girlfriend talked an awful lot about how she *saw* their relationship, whereas he preferred to *discuss* things. 'Wow, this is something that could really prove useful in strengthening our relationship,' Joe said to himself, his inner voice suddenly more confident.

Richard, too, had found it useful:

So, in the first books we set out to design patterns that everybody would be able to learn. Everybody could learn to listen to what Virginia did and to ask the same questions as she did. In fact, you will learn more about it this afternoon. Is that correct, Alan?

All heads turned. At the back of the room, Alan nodded with a knowing smile.

Now, back in the Santa Cruz Mountains, one of my neighbours was an Englishman named Gregory Bateson.

A brilliant man, very much of an intellectual, very well known, Gregory had read my first book – actually he had found it so interesting that he had ended up writing the introduction – and one day he said to me, 'Richard, there's something you need to do!'

'What is it, Gregory?'

'You have to go to Arizona and meet Milton H. Erickson.'

'Who's Milton Erickson?'

'Oh, he's a medical doctor and a very famous therapist! I've sent people over to see what he's doing and no one has even remembered being there.'

'Cool! That's something I might like!'

So we shot down to Arizona to meet with this guy who was

considered – with every reason – to be one of the greatest therapists alive. We watched Milton work with clients, and when we got back, we wrote a book explaining how he used language.

See, Milton stood out for me for three reasons. First, he was the one to theorize that the unconscious was always listening and that you could communicate at different levels of understanding even in what appeared to be a regular conversation.

Second, Milton realized that feelings were contagious. That means if you want someone to feel good, you have to begin by going into a wonderful state yourself.

Last, what was really admirable about Milton was that no matter how crazy somebody was, he never looked at being 'crazy' as something for which you should be incarcerated forever, and he never looked at drugs as being the answer to making stupid decisions.

Milton and Virginia never gave up on people. When Virginia started working with somebody, she didn't stop until they changed. Period. It didn't matter to her if it took one hour or 25 – when she got it into her mind that someone could change, she would simply never stop. Milton was very much the same, and I got that from them. That kind of relentless determination is absolutely necessary to be effective at what we do.

Now, what NLP is all about is the promotion of what I like to call *personal freedom*. It means your ability to choose how you handle your brain, your behaviour and your life. But before we dive into this, let's take a ten-minute break.

Joe took the chance to get a coffee, then returned to his seat and resumed his conversation with Edgar.

'So, you were telling me about Alan …'

'Oh, yes. I've found him to be an exceptional trainer. He's like the Obi-Wan Kenobi of NLP. The force is strong with him. LOL.'

He actually said the letters 'L O L' out loud! Joe couldn't believe it. It was all he could do not to cringe.

Oblivious, Edgar continued, 'Right from the start he gave me the feeling that he knew what he was talking about and, most importantly, he knew how to get it across. It's as though he always knows exactly where the audience is and how to capture their attention: giving an extra example at the right time, cracking a joke here and there, showing how the different ideas and techniques work together to create a seamless process.' Edgar put on a squeaky high voice to sound like Yoda from *Star Wars* and added, 'How to use the good side of the force, understand he does.'

Joe couldn't help laughing. Edgar *was* actually funny – in his own, very unique way.

'I never had the pleasure of seeing him onstage,' he replied, 'but I can relate to what you're saying. Having someone like him as one of the assistants on the previous course really made a difference. He helped me to clear my doubts whenever I had them.'

It was then that Joe noticed, out of the corner of his eye, that Emily seemed to be pretty down. Her mother had gone out for a moment and she was just sitting motionless in her seat, her right hand cupped over her eyes. Just as Joe was about to excuse himself and see if she was OK, Teresa returned to her seat. Immediately Emily plastered a huge smile on her face.

It was none of Joe's business, but he wanted to find out what was up with Emily. He vowed to keep an eye on her.

Chapter 3

HOW TO FEEL GOOD

After the break, Richard returned promptly to the stage.

Now, probably one of the most important lessons I learned in studying Virginia and Milton was that they always focused on getting the client into a different emotional state when thinking about their problems.

If they could get the client to think about the problem while feeling good, it helped them to make powerful changes.

NLP was created to give people more control over their mind. That's in essence what we're doing here. You have to realize that you can create any state that you want, whenever you want. You can learn to look at the same piece of personal history in a different way … Because the truth is that it's not your personal history that makes you who you are, it's your response to it.

This was a particularly important concept for Joe. *It's not my past that makes me who I am but how I respond to it.* He considered this while Richard continued:

> Everything I've done in the last 40 years has been about having personal freedom — that is, the freedom of choice. I don't want to make it so that you can't get angry or scared anymore. I want to make sure you can choose *when* to get angry or scared and *what* to get angry or scared about. That way, you can begin to make all of these things useful. Fear keeps you safe and out of trouble, but a fear of elevators? Really?
>
> You should be terrified of things that are worth being afraid about, like wasting your life mulling over the past!

Joe knew that recently he hadn't been getting on as well with his girlfriend partly because he was feeling under pressure, and that something similar was happening to her. *I need to take more control over my moods*, he thought.

> Now, the first thing that I want you to do today is a thought experiment.
>
> Whenever we think, we do so in three primary ways: we create mental images and movies, we talk to ourselves and we have feelings.
>
> Now, for years everyone was asking about *what* happened in your life rather than *how* you were thinking about it. What I discovered was that *the way* you thought about things was what determined how you felt. What that means is that you can help

people change when you teach them to take control of the movies they make in their mind and the way they talk to themselves.

I guess everybody here goes to the movies at least once in a while, so you might be familiar with the sensation of seeing a film on the big screen and actually enjoying it, then seeing it again some time later on a small TV set and not finding it half as good as you remembered it.

Joe knew exactly what Richard was talking about. In fact, he had recently seen a movie on TV and it hadn't just looked worse – even the story had made less sense than it had at the cinema!

That is because the size of the picture matters when it comes to feeling more or less involved. Even if the content remains the same, when you change the quality of the picture – its size, brightness, distance and colour – your whole experience changes.

Now, think of something that happened to you recently and still bothers you, something that you wish to have off your mind …

An episode came to Joe's mind: an argument he had had with a drunk guy who had been hitting on his girlfriend a couple of nights back.

Chances are that you are imagining a life-size scene as vividly as if you were actually there, right?

When Joe thought about it, it was true: he was remembering the event as if it was a movie playing in front of him.

Take that picture and begin by making it smaller. Then move it off into the distance and drain the colour out of it. If you hear the voices and sounds of the scene, make them fade away together with the brightness. Make the picture so small you have to squint to see what's in there, and then make it even smaller. When it's the size of a breadcrumb, you can just brush it away – just like that.

Joe followed the instructions to the letter. As he made the picture smaller, he also made the sound of the guy's voice quieter and imagined the picture moving further and further away. As he did so, he started to feel far better about the experience.

That feels better, right?

Almost everyone nodded.

Good. Then I suggest you leave it where it is!
See, this is the point where people usually ask me, 'And what if it comes back?' Well, if it does, you just take ten more seconds of your time – it really shouldn't take more than that – and do it again. After you have done it a few times, your brain will get the hang of it and start doing it all by itself.
And since we're talking about it, let me show you another way to make a positive change stick. This time I want you to think of

something fun. I know some of you are more used to thinking of something awful, but it's never too late. It's actually incredible: you ask an audience to think of something terrible and they all have it right away. Then you ask them to think of something fun … well, let me put it like this: some of you take this whole fun business dead seriously!

So, I want you guys to think of something fun-tastic and then together we'll explore your personal control room. That's the place where the magic happens and you can shape things just the way you want to.

Imagine a screen right in front of you, so you can see whatever you want to there.

Now, think back to a really pleasant experience, one where you really had a good time. That's *really* had a good time – if it doesn't make you feel like giggling even now, it's not what you're looking for.

See what you saw at the time, hear what you heard and feel what you felt. Really imagine you're back there and it's happening now.

Joe remembered a boat trip he had been on recently with his girlfriend. He remembered how both of them had been in stitches over a funny face Joe had made at her. It had been such an amazing afternoon he started to beam just thinking about it. Meanwhile, a woman in one of the front rows erupted in quite distinctive laughter. Richard looked down at her.

That's right, you obviously got my meaning! And when the rest of you find a memory that's that good, hold that thought for a spell.

Now, what I want you to do is imagine a lever that says 'Fun' and slowly move it up. To make it feel even more real, actually make the gesture. That's right.

I know some of you feel that this is a ridiculous thing to do. Here's my advice for you: do the exercise. Imagine that lever, grab it, and when you get to the point where you really feel that it's a stupid thing to do, consider this: *the things that you do that make your life unpleasant are even stupider.*

As Joe remembered the boat trip vividly, a huge grin appeared on his face. As the wonderful feeling spread throughout his body, he imagined grabbing a lever and starting to move it up.

Now, as you allow the image of the exhilarating memory to get closer and closer and bigger and brighter, start slowly sliding the lever up, only at the rate and speed that fits the changes in your physiology. Allow that exhilarating memory to get closer and closer and bigger and brighter. Add colour to the image of the memory, make it shine, look at the details ...

And as you do this, hear a voice in your head saying, 'Let the fun begin.'

Joe could feel himself taking off as the movie got bigger and more vivid and he moved the lever up.

This is an NLP technique we call 'anchoring.' You take a sensation and associate it with a stimulus – in this case the lever in the control panel of your mind. Since the two things came together, your brain decides they must belong together. This wonderful technique allows you to capture any feeling and associate it with an internal image like the lever, or a touch, or a word, or a movement; that way you can use that stimulus later to retrigger that feeling when you need it.

Joe found himself feeling really, really good as Richard gave everyone a few moments to enjoy their inner movies before saying:

OK, now come back to Earth. I want to show you something. You don't need to take time to create these feelings in the future because you have your lever. So, now that most of you are back on planet Earth, try this: in your mind, close your eyes and just grab hold of that lever again and move it up as you say to yourself, 'Let the fun begin.'

Joe tried it, and the exhilarating sensation came right back. He was looking forward to practising this!

This is how anchors work in NLP. The number of hours most people spend feeling bad is absolutely ridiculous and the number of hours when you haven't immersed yourself in enjoying the magic of being alive, because you were too busy, is crazy. I know these are hectic times, but if you're going to rush anyway, you might as well enjoy it. You can make every single thing you do magical, especially when you're with other people: just remember to go into the right state.

The question I get people to ask themselves is, 'How good can you feel for no reason whatsoever?' And if you think that's a crazy notion, think about this: people actually relive arguments that they didn't have! Isn't that weird? And they don't even do it for fun; they do it to make themselves feel bad. They have imaginary arguments and they go through them over and over again in their head.

Listen to this: a woman − a perfectly intelligent human being with a PhD and everything − came into my office and told me, 'I've been in therapy for 16 years, and still I argue with my mother all the time.'

'Where's your mother?' I asked.

'My mother is dead.'

Now, I don't know about you, but that gave me the willies.

'And you argue with her all the time.'

'Inside my head,' she specified, as if that would make it somewhat better.

I've been to many places in my life, seen lots of weird things, but I've never heard spookier things than what people tell me about the inside of their mind. The idea that somebody would spend hours upon hours arguing with a dead person inside their head … In fact, I asked her, 'Did it never occur to you just not to do this?'

She looked at me as if I was nuts. And she's sitting there having arguments with her mother, back and forth, instead of having a life!

See, there's a real difference between the inside and the outside of your mind, and you should understand that it's your brain and you can make it do what you want it to. You just need to be able to realize that the voices inside your head have volume controls. You can make them louder, you can make them softer, you can make them say what you want to – and in whatever tone of voice you choose.

As Joe jotted down what Richard had just said, his mind went back to his girlfriend and to the first time they had met. How different his life would be now, if back then he hadn't taken control of that nagging voice in his own head. But now it was getting out of control and jeopardizing his entire relationship. He had to get back to basics and refuse to let it dictate his thoughts and feelings the way it had been doing lately.

And now I want to tell you about this. A group of people – and don't ask me how they had this idea – they took a yoghurt culture, divided it in half and attached half of it to something that could measure its electrical activity.

Then they poured milk over the other half – you know, that's what yoghurt eats: milk.

Now, when this half got fed, the other half – the one with the sensors – began to respond: it knew the other half was being fed!

So they asked me, 'Richard, how can we explain that when we feed the yoghurt over here, the other half knows?'

'Because they're twins!'

'Well, that's not much of an explanation.'

'Well, there's another simple explanation, then: yoghurt knows yoghurt.'

They looked at me totally confused, but I believe that everything is alive in its own way. Even ideas are alive. That's what makes this so important.

Next the researchers tried to put walls between the two halves of the yoghurt. They made them out of wood, they made them out of different metals, they tried electromagnetic barriers, and still when they fed one half of the yoghurt, the other half went wild.

They said, 'We just don't understand. There has to be an explanation for this.'

I told them that there was one and that if they left me alone there, I would build a wall the yoghurt couldn't communicate through.

They said, 'It's impossible, Richard. We've tried everything.'

And I went, 'No, you haven't.'

But that's what happens when you mistake your map for the territory it's supposed to describe. When people refuse to accept that reality might be somewhat more complex and varied than their representation of it, they have no space left for improvement.

When these guys came back, one week later, I had built the barrier. They did the experiment and the yoghurt didn't respond, so they asked, 'What is this barrier made of?' The truth is, it was a fish tank full of yoghurt. Because when one of the yoghurts vibrated into the yoghurt wall, the vibration was absorbed. It could only go so far.

This is why it is so important for you to realize that the state you're in is the primary tool you're working with. You can't be depressed and expect to help people be cheerful.

As it turned out, when I built the wall out of yoghurt, I understood that things that vibrate vibrate together. When you pluck a piano string, all of the strings with that harmonic will vibrate. It's just that things know each other. Which means that if you go around grumpy, you will meet grumpy people, or people will be grumpy around you. You reap what you sow.

Yoghurt knows yoghurt and people know people. If you want someone to feel a certain way, you have to go there first.

Hearing this, it suddenly occurred to Joe that his emotional states definitely affected his girlfriend in a big way. Whenever he came home from work stressed and she came over, he found her becoming more and more irritated as the night went on. *Well, perhaps those big mood changes aren't about her at all. Perhaps it's my state that affects her*, he thought. This was quite a revelation.

Richard was talking about the difference states could make:

For example, I worked with this guy who was head of a company. His problem was that he was scared of meeting women. The crazy thing was that when I asked what he did as a hobby, he said, 'Ski-jumping.'

'The one where you jump off the side of a mountain and fly through the air?'

'Yes,' he said.

'And you're scared of women?'

'Yep!'

'Sure,' I indulged him, 'they can be pretty scary. Especially when they fight over that last pair of shoes on sale!'

Everyone laughed.

This is where you try to make people feel as stupid as they're acting. Because if people *don't* feel as stupid as they're acting, they'll start to take their problems too seriously. And if you take problems too seriously, then you just make them more real, because, you see, these things *aren't* real, they're illusions. Stepping on a nail that goes through your foot – that's real, and it hurts, yet people can learn to control even that pain.

Anyhow, this guy told me that when he looked at women, he became absolutely petrified. So I looked at him and I said, 'OK, let me get this straight: you put a pair of sticks on your feet, wax them up, slide down a mountain at a really fast speed, shoot off the mountain and into space, flying through the air for hundreds of yards without a parachute … and this doesn't scare you?'

'No, it's exhilarating.'

'And you see a person sitting by herself at a table, drinking coffee. And to walk over and say hello frightens you.'

'Yeah, absolutely.'

'Jumping off a mountain … versus saying hello. It doesn't balance out to me somehow.'

And he looked at me sheepishly and said, 'I know it sounds nuts.'

'That's because it is!' I told him. 'Let's turn this around. You know that feeling of exhilaration you get right before you jump?'

'Yes, yes!'

'OK. Take that feeling and spin it in your body. Make it stronger and stronger. Now, I want you to go downstairs and, as you spin that feeling, I want you to just walk up to people and say hello. Find the people that you would never talk to. If you start to feel afraid, all I want you to do is to simply remember the feeling you have just before you jump off a mountain. Because, you know, this is going to help you, whereas feeling afraid is not. So, if you start to feel afraid, just stop. Stop thinking about it, go back, remember the feeling of exhilaration, then look at what you want to do and take that feeling with you.

So he went out and he was gone for about an hour. I finally sent somebody down to look for him, and when they came back, they told me, 'He won't come back because he's talking to a lady!'

Joe laughed. It was like the first time he had met his girlfriend. He remembered talking to himself continuously about how she wouldn't be interested in getting to know him. *How strange*, he thought, *that someone I'm now so comfortable with used to be someone I was terrified of talking to.*

Now, let me demonstrate how you can take the good feelings that we anchored before and use them to transform your life. Excuse me, ma'am, what's your name?

Richard was pointing down to the woman Joe had seen rummaging anxiously through her bag earlier. *This should be interesting*, he thought. *Quite a challenge.*

The woman looked more stressed than ever as Richard pointed at her. Her face went bright red. 'Liz,' she replied in a strained voice.

What do you do, Liz? When you're not worrying, that is?

Liz seemed shocked that he knew. Richard just smiled.

Don't be so surprised, Liz, it was written all over your face. Literally. Do you know when you screw your face up like that it's not conducive to really good feelings?

Liz shook her head.

Well, when you smile your brain releases happy chemicals into your body and when you frown it releases a different set of chemicals that produce stress and worry. A good idea would be to relax your face more and give yourself a dose of good feelings.

So, what do you do, Liz?

'I'm a teacher,' she said, just loud enough for Joe to hear.

A teacher? Well now, it's more important than ever that you get this right, Liz. Because yoghurt knows yoghurt and the children in

40

your class need to be around the right kind of yoghurt – the healthy type, if you get my meaning.

But before I invite Liz onto the stage let's take a five-minute break.

Joe was looking forward to seeing how this would work out with Liz. It would be interesting to see if Richard could help her. He looked over his notes and after a few minutes Richard continued:

Now, Liz, can you come up here and help me out with something? You look far too stressed and I want to teach you a technique that can help you.

Liz made her way to the stage and sat down beside Richard. She was panting almost audibly.

Let me ask you a question, Liz: how much time do you spend feeling bad?

'Hours and hours,' she replied meekly.

Joe almost laughed out loud at the honesty of this lady. To admit that you spent lots of your day feeling bad seemed funny to him. But the disturbing thing was that he had been spending a little too much time doing the very same thing himself. He knew he had to pay attention to what Richard was saying.

Glad to see you're being straight with me, Liz. The thing I want you to consider is this: when you change, what are you going to do with all that time? Just think about all the spare time you'll have. *That's* what I worry about! Some of you guys spend so much time worrying and fretting that you can't even remember how to feel really great any longer. If I only tackle what troubles you, chances are you'll just find something else to fuss about. That's why we are going to do things my way.

I have a recommendation, and some of you might want to try it. I want you to close your eyes, Liz, and I want you to think about one of the best feelings you've ever had.

Richard paused, allowing her to access the experience. She frowned in concentration, obviously struggling with the recollection.

Try something so good you can't possibly tell us about it.

Liz blushed, her frown melting into a smile.

That's it! That's what I'm talking about. See, guys, the right thought can affect your entire physiology instantly. That's just how powerful the mind is. This is the kind of response you want to elicit and enhance, so that you can use it every day to make your life absolutely fantastic.

OK, now this feeling, this really amazing feeling, tell me, where does it start in your body? What part of you? And where does it move to?

HOW TO FEEL GOOD

Liz thought for a while and then answered, 'My stomach. It moves up.'

Up, OK. Now, when the good feeling goes away, where does it go? When you stop thinking about that feeling, where does it go?

After a few seconds, Liz pushed her hands away from her body. 'Out,' she responded.

OK, here's a little trick that will really help you out: let the good feeling come up, and just before it goes away, pull it out and back to the beginning, so that it moves in a circle, and begin to spin it round and round.
That's right.

Liz began to smile as she started concentrating again.

Spin it faster as you keep thinking about that experience. And faster. That's right.
Now even it out, so it spins in the middle as it spins around even faster. See, you have no idea how much pleasure your body is capable of.
Spin it faster, and if you keep spinning it, it's going to change in a very unique way.

The tension on Liz's face was dissipating – she even chuckled.

That's right, feel free to enjoy yourself – while changing your life for good.

Of course, you do realize that the faster you spin the feeling and the faster it goes around, the sooner there's a point at which it feels really good? That's when people are going to stop you and say, 'What happened to you? You're smiling all the time. What's wrong with you?' I love it when they do that. Then you just look at them and laugh.

And that's exactly what Liz did. In fact Joe noticed her mood was rapidly spreading through the audience. *Richard's right*, he thought. *States are contagious.*

Richard was explaining further:

You see, if it's a good feeling, you don't want it to go away – you just want it to build up, to stay there and get stronger.

Even better, we're going to take this good feeling and we're going to add something to it, because I know you'll face situations in the future that have made you feel bad in the past.

Now I'd like to tell you about a technique you can use to banish bad feelings. OK, Liz?

Liz nodded.

What I want you to do is to think about the very thing that made you feel bad. Just imagine watching it on a screen and taking hold of the brightness dial. Then, in one quick move, I want you to turn that dial all the way to bright, so you completely white the picture out – one moment you see it, and the next it's just completely whited out.

As Liz did this, she jerked slightly in the chair.

Excellent! Do it again. Imagine the thing that made you feel bad. Now white it out, real quick. And again. And again. Now, take that really good feeling that you were spinning, and as you imagine that situation in the future, white out the bad thought and spin this really good feeling around.

As you do this, you're going to hear an inner voice that says, 'Never again!'

Because sometimes you're going to feel that enough is enough and you're not going to allow yourself to keep on doing it. If you think about the number of hours you've wasted on this and think about how much fun you can have instead, you won't spend your time doing things that you don't want to do anymore. That's how you'll have time to create new, positive habits.

So, imagine yourself in this difficult situation in the future, but this time, white out any negative image and feel this good feeling spinning faster throughout your body – and notice what happens.

Now ... I want you to stop and think about that situation and see how you feel about it. Can you imagine feeling bad?

Liz tried, but her face only showed surprise, then relaxed aware-ness that a change had actually occurred.

The truth is that if you go into the right state, you can do just about anything, but if you don't change your own internal state, then how can you expect anything else to change?

When I started out, being an information scientist, I went about things differently than everyone else. I went and put an ad in the newspaper, asking for people who used to have phobias and got rid of them. I had about 100 people come in and I said to each one, 'OK, you had a phobia. How did you get rid of it?'

And they all told me basically the same story. It went something like: 'Well, after years and years, I got so fed up with it I said, "That's it. I can't take it anymore. That was the straw that broke the camel's back."' And then they all stopped, slapped their forehead and said, 'At that moment, I looked at myself and I saw how stupid it was to be afraid.'

1. And I wrote down the following:
2. Slap forehead (probably optional!)
3. Disassociate – that is, see yourself in the image

Watch yourself doing it from a dissociated point of view

And I decided to try it out on people who still had phobias.

At that time there was this guy from Wessington. His problem was that he had panic attacks every time he tried to leave town.

So I asked him to imagine driving toward the edge of town and to observe the scene as if he were Superman flying next to his vehicle, looking at himself driving his pick-up truck. As he was flying, he watched himself skid to a halt, get out of the truck and freak out, but the part of him that was observing the whole scene just flew on, right out of town. Now, the trick is that inside his mind I already had him calmly flying and, at the same time, I had him out of town.

Now, if you see yourself from a distance sitting in the front seat of a roller-coaster, it's a totally different experience than actually sitting there. It's a different perspective and a different set of feelings. Knowing that these things are different, when people want to change their feelings, one of the things I've always done is to find a way they could literally get a new perspective.

And this brings us back to the thought experiment we tried before. This change of perspective is just another of those variables – together with the brightness or the size of the picture – that you find in people's minds. In NLP we call them *submodalities*.

And now, let's give Liz a round of applause. Thank you, Liz.

And with that, Liz went back to her seat looking a lot better than she had when she had staggered onstage a few minutes before.

Joe was intrigued as Richard explained more about submodalities:

Let me go over this idea one more time. Inside your head, pictures have to have a place, they have to have a distance, they have to have a size; they're either in black and white or they're in colour, they're a movie or they're a slide. Sounds have to come from the right and/or from the left; they sound either like they're going in or like they're going out. These, to me, seem to be the important distinctions that we have to make about things. That should be in our owner's manual. Unfortunately, we don't come with one, so we have to create our own.

The reason why I concentrate so much at this point on finding out where feelings start and how they move – and on making the pictures smaller or bigger and the feelings go backward – is that I discovered the simplest thing of all, which is that you can repattern your behaviour by changing the way you feel. And you can change the way you feel by doing something different with the sounds and images you make inside your mind.

Now, I had Liz come up here, and she sat down for what – five minutes or so?

As Richard looked at Liz, she nodded and smiled brightly. She looked much more relaxed.

In your mind, you took something and whited it out, and you ran your good feelings faster, didn't you? And when you think about it now, it feels totally different.

And this is serious business, right, Liz?

Richard's voice sounded grave and worried. He looked sternly at Liz – who burst out laughing!

Hey, what are you laughing for? What about your problems? Where are the pain and suffering? Oh, I see: you're resisting change! Do you want your problem back? You see, the trouble is that because I don't need to know what the problem is in the first place, I don't ask. And then, when people want their problem back, I risk giving them back the wrong problem.

Liz was holding her belly now, her face turning red with laughter, as Richard continued:

Think about all those things that made you feel bad. Come on, you can do it! All the thoughts that made you feel stressed, worried, anxious …

Liz was laughing louder and louder.

It can't be this easy. You need to spend lots more time feeling bad. You can't be feeling better already! Liz, you really are a terrible client. What about all the mistakes you made? What about your bad experiences?

She just kept laughing, and as she did so, the crowd started up as well. Richard looked at the audience and winked, his eyes twinkling.

Wouldn't it be awful if every time you started to feel bad, you just got a rush of the giggles? Because to me, the real trick is to go inside and change the images in your mind and the way you talk to yourself and make your brain feel really good. This is what I refer to as 'ridiculous therapy'!

When I did it with the client who had a fear of women, he was able to change the way he behaved. He wasn't able to approach a woman until something inside him made it fun. You can only do that by taking the things that appear difficult and changing the way you feel about them. And this isn't done by rummaging around in your childhood. If your childhood messed you up, going back to it is just going to mess you up more.

Since we are speaking about childhood, it's time that you gave a little of *this good* feeling to the children in your class, Liz. Tell me, have you ever noticed that when you're in a bad mood, things seem harder and even a little problem can feel like the end of the world? Do you think it's possible that when you feel bad, it rubs off on the children? Have you noticed that when you feel good you can handle the class much more easily?

Liz, her face now shining, paused for a second, then responded, 'Yes, sometimes I get out of bed on the wrong side in the morning and I just know the children are going to be difficult ...'
Richard interrupted her:

Has it ever occurred to you that maybe, just maybe, it's not about you having psychic powers and being able to predict how they'll be? What if, instead, you deliberately decided to feel good for absolutely no reason whatsoever? How do you think your students would respond to you if you were in a good mood more often? Think about it. Teaching might just be easier.

Liz contemplated this for a moment with a frown, as if she were considering the possibility that it was actually *her* mood that influenced the children and not the other way around. Then it looked as if she suddenly had a lightbulb moment, which is when Richard added:

> Either that or just move your bed against the wall. Then you can only get out of it on the right side.

That started Liz laughing again. Richard turned to the audience:

> Now, it's about time you all got a chance to try this out. Pick a partner, introduce yourself, then get to it. Decide who's going to go first. Then ask the other person whether there's a part of their life where they feel stuck or blocked, a situation where they get bad feelings every time and this limits their behaviour, because it leads to the most horrible thing human beings can do: hesitate. And hesitate and hesitate, and the next thing they know is that there's no opportunity left. Because when opportunity passes you by, you can watch it walk into the distance and then live in regret for the rest of your life, or you can jump on it and try some things.

Joe stirred in his chair. He couldn't wait to get up and do the exercise right away. But Richard had a few more instructions first:

> I want you to sit down with the partner you pick and have them go into a state where they feel really good. Now, the key is for you to go first. Remember – yoghurt knows yoghurt. So …

1. Go inside and think of something that makes you feel really wonderful. Make the image big and vivid to increase the feelings.
2. Two, get your partner to do the very same thing. Have them spin the good feeling all the way through their body until they feel amazing.
3. Have them think of the troubling time in the future and have them think of what makes them feel bad. Have them grab that brightness dial and white it out. Do this two or three times really fast.
4. Get them to spin the really wonderful feeling throughout their body so that they are filled with an incredible sense of well-being.

When you do all that, you'll enable them to change how they think about the situation and you'll give them what really matters: the freedom to feel as good as they want when they need it the most.

Now get on with it.

Even though he had overcome a certain degree of romantic shyness in his personal life, by now Joe was fully aware he hadn't been using some of the same skills at work. Whenever he thought about certain meetings, he would go inside and worry about what would happen if he made a fool of himself or forgot what he was talking about. He no longer felt scared of presenting; it was more that he felt uncomfortable when he was talking to certain people individually. If they were strangers, he felt that he was boring them. He decided to work with Teresa on this issue.

Teresa started by getting in the right state herself, then turned to Joe and had him go inside his mind and think about a time he felt really, really good. Joe thought about a weekend where he had gone away with his girlfriend and they had had the best fun ever. He had laughed more on that weekend than he had in a long time.

When Joe was smiling brightly, Teresa had him double the size of the movie and imagine it even more vividly. Joe started beaming. Then Teresa had him spin the good feeling all the way through his body.

Next, Teresa had Joe think of a time in the future that he was concerned about. He thought about a specific meeting that was coming up in a couple of weeks. But before he had a chance to get nervous, Teresa asked him to imagine the brightness dial and turn it all the way up, so that he could white out the image. He did this a few times and then she had him spin the good feeling around again.

At the end, Teresa suggested that Joe think about the future meeting. He smiled. He was feeling far better about it. At that moment a thought occurred to him: *If it felt so good just doing this once, how much better would it become through practising it on a regular basis, imagining different situations?* Maybe shyness wasn't a fixed personality trait. *Maybe,* he considered, *shyness is just a state of mind.*

Then they swapped and Joe helped Teresa with her own issue. Despite having successfully applied NLP in her life and in her work as a doctor, Teresa explained that she struggled when it came to handling difficult people. When she dealt with particularly aggressive individuals she lost confidence in herself.

Joe, who was already feeling incredibly good from having gone through the process, had Teresa think of how she felt when she was at her most confident and got her to spin the feeling through her body. Next, as she beamed, he had her make an image of having to deal with an aggressive person in the future. He got her to white out the image and had her imagine the good feeling spinning around her body. To his delight, as he brought her through the process, Teresa's entire body straightened up and by the end she was looking substantially more confident.

Richard came back onstage.

How did you do? Pretty fun, huh? When you started thinking of very pleasant things, didn't the other person start smiling? That means there's something infectious going on. Humans influence one another every time they communicate, and building good feelings shouldn't just be something you do here, but be a part of how you do things every day. When you think about your marriage, you should associate it with every good memory you have, and when you think about unpleasant things – well, just stay out of the picture. If you associate your marriage with every bad thing your spouse does, you'll be angry with them all the time.

If you happen to think about an unpleasant thing that has happened to you in your life, make sure it looks like a black-and-white Polaroid, then push it off into the distance and pretty soon it won't matter so much.

If you vibrate all kinds of things such as happiness, joy, excitement ... well, guess what? People around you will start doing just the same without even knowing what happened. If you can go into a state that feels good, people around you will do the same. These are the things that your unconscious is taking in.

Now let's have lunch. Be back in an hour and a half feeling great and ready for a surprise!

Richard left the stage to a big round of applause.

Joe, Teresa and Emily left together, and Joe asked Edgar to join them. As they sat down in the restaurant, Joe shared something that had been on his mind all day: 'This morning, Teresa, you said something about certainty preventing learning that I didn't quite understand. Surely having strong beliefs and certainties is a good thing?'

'I suppose we could say that it's not certainty *per se* that's bad,' Teresa clarified. 'There are things that it's good to be certain about and there are times when being certain becomes an obstacle.'

'I'm still confused about it,' Joe admitted.

'That's exactly what I mean. Now that you have heard that the map isn't the territory, let me put it this way: if you came here and experienced no confusion whatsoever, it would mean that you had managed to fit everything you saw and heard into your old map. Some people feel so certain that their map *is* the territory that no matter what information comes in they'll manage to fit it into what they already know.'

While Teresa was speaking, Joe noticed the expression on Emily's face. She wasn't really listening to them, just looking off into the distance. Something was troubling her, but it seemed that she didn't want her mother to notice. As Joe caught her eye, she immediately checked herself and turned away, a little embarrassed.

'Look, Joe,' Teresa continued, 'it's like trying to fit a square peg in a round hole. If you hold on to your certainty that the map *is* the territory, you will automatically assume that all pegs must be round. Then you can only make sense of what you're experiencing in one of two ways: you either "distort" the square peg until you manage to fit it into a round hole or you discard it as not relevant, thus "deleting" that piece of evidence. In either case, certainty serves only to reinforce the belief that you are right about things. It's doubt that makes space for creating a hole that fits the square peg just fine. So, I think that "no confusion" could mean "no learning". You can't find out something new about yourself or the world without modifying or expanding your map. And you don't change your map without at least a slight sense of confusion. Confusion is the doorway to clarity.'

'And if you look at what Richard is doing onstage,' Edgar added, 'it's true that he's having us build strong beliefs, but he's also taking quite a lot of time and energy to bring down the typical beliefs that hold people back, like the idea that change must be slow and painful.'

'You guys seem to have it all figured out,' Joe said with a touch of envy.

'Grey hair must count for something!' Edgar joked.

'By the way,' Joe asked, 'how do you integrate psychotherapy and NLP?'

'Easily!' Edgar chipped back.

'I mean, don't you have to struggle to put the two things together?'

'Not at all. NLP offers some very remarkable tools to understand how we communicate with ourselves and with the rest of the world. You can apply those tools in lots of different contexts. That's why NLP is so appealing to people from all walks of life, I guess.'

'And how did you get to NLP?' Teresa asked Edgar.

'Working in my profession, sooner or later you're bound to hear about Richard Bandler's work. Personally, I'm always looking for new points of view, new approaches, new techniques that I can add to my own set of tools. Whenever I get stuck with a client, I know it's time to explore something new. That keeps me open to new possibilities. I'm curious by nature and having a challenge helps me stay motivated. I've learned a lot from the field of NLP. One thing I always remind myself of – especially when I see "bad" behaviour – is another important NLP principle: *people make the best choice they can at the time.* That means that a person often makes the best choice they can, given their map of the world. The choice may be self-defeating or bizarre, but for them it seems the best way forward. Help them expand their map of the world and they will make better choices.'

Joe liked this concept a lot. Thinking about how to apply it in his life, he considered the idea that it was essential to understand and respect the map of others. *My map*, he thought, *represents how I think of the world and determines what I do and how I communicate with others. If a co-worker operates from a map that is significantly different from mine, it might be difficult to communicate with that person. We won't understand each other very well.*

Joe decided that from now on he was going to step back and learn more about his colleagues' points of view and perspectives.

While he was considering this, Emily joined the conversation: 'So, when I fail miserably to get through to one of my friends about something, is that because their map is different from mine? Sometimes I feel, as the saying goes, that *everyone is wise until they speak.*'

Joe grinned. Emily was quite a character. From this teenager's mouth came pearls of wisdom he would have expected to hear from a wise 80-year-old man in a pub in the heart of Dublin.

Teresa also smiled. 'Yes, dear. It's because of the difference between your maps. And here's a thought that might prove useful in situations like that: what if the meaning of your communication wasn't what you intended, but the response you got?'

Emily gave her a perplexed look.

'It's one of the principles of NLP,' Edgar clarified. 'In order to make your communication more effective, you measure it on the response that you get. That way, if you get the response you wished for, your communication was successful, whereas if you get a different response, you still have the chance to succeed by changing what you're doing.'

'What you're saying,' Emily tried to summarize, 'is that it's not about the other person getting my meaning right as much as it is about me making myself understood?'

'I guess that could be one way of putting it,' Edgar confirmed. Then he looked at Teresa. 'What do you say?'

'I agree,' replied Teresa. 'And as long as you have this attitude, you can never fail at communicating, because the other person's response becomes the feedback that lets you know if you're heading in the right direction. That of course means you've got to take responsibility for your communication, and if you're not getting the result you want, you need to change what you're doing.'

Edgar agreed. 'The principle here is that people can never read your mind – except the Jedi, of course.'

Teresa chuckled along at this one.

Edgar continued, 'Of course people can make some educated guesses, but eventually they can respond only to what they *think* you mean, which may or may not be an accurate interpretation of your intended meaning. In my profession the value of this is that it points out that if we want people to respond appropriately to what we say, we need to talk *to* them rather than *at* them. That means we need to be constantly aware of other people's responses to what we're saying and adjust our communication accordingly, rather than just assuming that they will have understood what we meant them to understand.'

Joe made a mental note of this as he tucked into his lunch. He was really enjoying himself. This was one of the things he liked the most about these courses – having the chance to share experiences and insights with other participants.

Chapter 4

HOW TO BECOME A MASTERFUL COMMUNICATOR

Before going back after lunch, Joe took a brief walk by himself to the nearby park. He wanted to capitalize on the exercise they had just done by thinking through as many of his work meetings as he could and practising changing his feelings about them.

Joe felt that he had learned some truly valuable ways of taking more control over how he felt. He already felt much more in charge of his life. He decided to experiment with his submodalities. In addition to working on the technique he had practised with Teresa, he tried to shrink the size of the negative images he made. This made them less intense. When he drained the colour from his negative thoughts, that helped as well. Since his critical inner voice still seemed to affect him negatively, he knew he had to do something about that as well. Instead of focusing on *what* he was saying, he worked on *how* he was saying it – the tone of voice he used when he criticized himself. Giving it a nicer sound actually made him feel a lot better.

Satisfied with the results, he proceeded back to the seminar room and found himself a place to sit. By the time Richard came onstage, he was smiling away, already looking forward to his next few meetings. Feeling better about them was an excellent start, but he knew he also needed to learn the most effective way of communicating with his clients and colleagues. He was full of anticipation as Richard began to speak:

Now, this morning you learned not only that you can take more control over how you feel but also that you affect others without even speaking to them. Your state affects their state – yoghurt knows yoghurt, remember.

This afternoon, I want to go for something different, because when we started out years ago with this stuff, we began by looking for what worked. Now, that wasn't just in therapy but in all aspects of communication. I began a process of building a model based on how the most successful salespeople, business leaders, teachers, doctors and therapists communicated.

What was interesting was that even if they operated in very different areas, the best communicators all had a number of things in common. They all had a powerful ability to create rapport with other people. They were able to communicate clearly, specifically and persuasively. They knew what questions to ask and how to make people feel really good.

As for the surprise I promised you earlier today, I'm going to ask Alan to come up here and teach you some basic skills of rapport and what we call *representational systems*. Alan is one of my best trainers, so please give him a big round of applause. I'll be back later.

Joe joined in the clapping as Alan made his way up to the stage. He was curious to see what he was like as a trainer. He smiled up at him. *He might need a friendly face*, he thought.

As Alan arrived onstage and shook Richard's hand, he appeared more confident than ever. As Richard left the stage, Alan thanked him, then began immediately:

Good afternoon, everyone. I expect you are well fed and ready for an exciting afternoon. So far you've learned how NLP can help you change the way you feel. Right now we're going to focus on how you can improve how you communicate with others.

When I started out a few years ago, well, let's just say I wasn't the best communicator around. I was often nervous around others and rarely made much of an impact. I let opportunities go by. I found it hard to connect with the people I met until I came across a number of really useful skills and tools on an NLP course.

It was hard for Joe to believe that Alan had once struggled with confidence. Fascinated, he looked up at him as Alan continued speaking:

The greatest thing I ever learned from NLP was that I had the ability to influence how well I got on with other people. I realized that you could actually become more likable, and this insight changed my life.

Anyway, let's start with building rapport with others. Rapport is a sense of connection that you create with others, a connection that makes both of you feel as if you understand each other well and have a lot in common. When two people get on really well together, they are known to be 'in rapport'.

Now, building rapport is a natural process. It happens all the time and we all do it to some degree or other. Call it what you will – rapport, empathy, being perceptive, tuning in – the bottom line is that we all do it.

Why am I telling you this? Because it's so natural that we end up considering it an inborn skill. Do you remember what people thought of Virginia Satir? That she was a miracle-worker. That her results weren't due to what she did but who she was. Luckily, someone was able to see beyond that, unveil the thinking and communication patterns behind her behaviour and model them so that those skills could be taught and learned.

As you know, NLP is largely about how to pay attention to what's going on around you. What Richard and his colleagues noticed was that when two people get on really well, they tend to match each other's communication patterns on all levels, verbal and non-verbal. The implications of this were exciting. They found that by deliberately matching another person's communication patterns, you could create a sense of profound connection with them.

Now, notice I'm not talking about mimicking. If you mirror a person's every move, they will very soon want to hit you in the face. 'Matching' means subtly and gradually adapting parts of your communication to be more in line with that of the other person. As I just said, this isn't only about verbal communication. The tone of your voice or the speed and tempo of your speech are also important. Also essential in order to establish rapport is your posture, including head movements, gestures, crossing or uncrossing your arms or legs and so forth.

Eager to check this out for himself, Joe looked around the seminar room. Sure enough, he found several examples of people sitting in exactly the same position. Take Teresa and Emily: they were both leaning forward with chin in hand, their head slightly tilted to one side.

In fact, one of the best things to match is a person's breathing. If you can breathe at the same rate as they do, that can be a powerful way of connecting with them. The more it remains out of their awareness, the better. In fact, the ultimate goal is to make it an unconscious process even for yourself – just like walking or driving a car. You want it to be a program that runs in the background, so you can focus on something else. And that will only come by practising these skills.

Once you get good at this, you can start to lead the other person into feeling and behaving as you do. This is called *pacing and leading*. So, if you are talking to a person who seems to be turned away and closed to you, once you pace them and gradually start to alter your body language to become more open, they will follow you with their own body language. It's just like …

Alan took a long, deep breath in and then exhaled slowly through his mouth. Then he stopped for a couple of seconds.

Joe couldn't help noticing that he himself did the very same thing.

When Alan asked how many in the audience had just taken a deeper breath, almost all hands went up. Alan's face lit up in a big smile as he resumed speaking.

That's what I'm talking about! See how naturally it happens?

Now, Richard asked me to show you the fine details about something he said earlier: rapport isn't only about your body or tone of voice, it's also about the language you use with others. In particular, when people communicate with you, they reveal how they are representing the world by the words that they use.

So, let's take a little step back for clarity. By now you have probably begun to recognize how our brain maps reality. We have five senses that we use to take information in from the world and so it makes sense that we have five ways to represent this information to ourselves. Basically it boils down to internal images, sounds and feelings, the other senses – smell and taste – being somewhat more limited in scope. In NLP, these modalities are better known as representational systems.

Richard has already given you a fine example of how Virginia Satir worked with these representational systems and has shown you how to take control of those representations by changing their submodalities – that is, the quality of the representation. What I'm saying here is that although all human beings experience the world through the same five senses, not everyone is aware of reality in the same way. Some of us prefer thinking in terms of visual images, others have a keen ear for sounds and words, and then there are those who rely primarily on bodily sensations to make sense of the world. Now, that doesn't mean we are that 'type' of person, but it does allow us to know how a person is thinking in a particular context.

Joe's thoughts went back to his relationship with his girlfriend. *She seems to really 'focus' a lot more on the visual aspects*, he thought. *It's incredible that I never noticed that before being told about these representational systems.*

Now, if you know what to look for and listen to, you're one step closer to understanding how people represent the world to themselves, and that, in turn, helps you build rapport at a much deeper level.

When people talk to us, they use sensory-related language, and the sensory words they use are clues they leave in language as to how they are thinking. For example, some people tend to use phrases such as 'the way it *looks* to me' or 'I *see* it differently' or 'in my *view*'. Others tend to use 'I *hear* what you are *saying*' or 'That *sounds* about right' or 'What you are *telling* me *resonates*.' And finally, there are people who say 'That *feels* right' or 'I get it and want to help you *grasp* it' or 'That *sits* well with me.'

Joe was scribbling furiously, adding these examples to the ones Richard had given in the morning when he had talked about Virginia Satir working with couples.

By listening to how a person speaks, you can identify how they are thinking, and that will help you to know how to communicate back to them. When they use visual words, *see* to it that you *show* them a *clear picture*. When they use auditory expressions, *tune in* and let yourself be *heard loud and clear*. When they use feeling words, *grasp* the chance to give them a *solid* understanding. This will help them feel that you are really speaking the same language as they are.

So, could someone describe to me their most recent holiday experience?

Joe heard Edgar's voice. 'Sure. I was in Rome recently. It was amazing. Such a beautiful place. Some of the structures are so big, but they have such a classic look to them. It was fantastic going around seeing the sights and spending time watching the people go about their business. I had a fantastic time. It really showed me that it is one of the prettiest cities around.'

Alan interrupted:

It does sound wonderful. Tell me, what were the people like to talk to?

Edgar looked slightly confused and stumbled. 'Eh, they were … I mean, nice, I suppose. They gesticulated so much I tended to get distracted by it!'

Some of the audience started to giggle. Alan continued:

Good. Some of you noticed what happened there. Edgar was describing things very visually. When I asked him about his auditory experience, it was hard for him to connect with that. Now, can I get another volunteer who can describe a holiday to me?

A lady in the front row called out, 'I've been to India, but I don't think in these representational systems.'
Alan smiled and said:

Everyone does to a degree. But let's hear your description anyway.

'Well,' she began, 'I was in India last month and what I loved about it was that I really connected with the place. It just felt so wonderful to be there. It was warm and a little sticky sometimes, but I just experienced so much contentment there.'
Alan interjected:

Wow, so did you get to grips with the culture? How did you connect with the local people? Did you feel comfortable there?

Without skipping a beat, the lady enthused, 'Oh, yes! It was really touching. I felt so welcome, as though it was my home. I really grasped the notion that India truly is a loving country with a big heart. I was so comfortable there.'
Again, some of the audience laughed. Joe understood why: this time, Alan had matched the representational system that

the lady was using. As she spoke in 'feeling' words, he had responded in kind, and that had helped move the conversation on effectively.

Alan went on with his explanation:

> When you match the representational system someone is using, it makes that person feel in rapport with you. When you 'mismatch' it, they don't feel as good — as you could see — because they're not hearing what resonates with them.

Joe noticed that Alan had used all three representational systems in that last sentence. What he said next explained why:

> Now, if you are speaking to a vast audience — such as this — and you want to match their favourite representational system, you actually need to use them all in turn. That will have two positive effects: it will help you establish rapport and it will give your audience a full sensory experience.
>
> But enough talking. It's direct experience time!
>
> Let's start with an exercise. I want you to get into groups of two. Person A will speak to person B, and person B will start by mismatching person A's body language while listening.
>
> Furthermore, person B will respond to something person A says, but will do so at a different rate of speech and will use a different representational system from person A.
>
> Meanwhile, person A will think about their experience and how they feel about person B.

Next, it's still person A talking to person B, but this time person B will subtly – and I mean *subtly* – match their body language, tone of voice, talking speed and representational systems.

Again, person A will think about their experience.

Then you will swap.

I'll see you back here in 15 minutes.

As Joe looked around for a partner, he made eye contact with an attractive woman in her early thirties. They decided to do the exercise together. She told him that her name was Caroline and that she was an actress.

'Hi, Caroline. I'm Joe. What brings you here?'

'Well, actually last year was a really tough year for me as I found out I had breast cancer. Going through that made me reconsider what I had been doing with my life. Now that I'm a lot better and have my life back, my dream is to become a professional actress. Along the way, I've been reading some books on personal development and self-help, and that's where I discovered NLP.'

'Wow, that's incredible. Congratulations on making it through all that.'

'Thanks, Joe. It was a long journey of pain but also self-discovery. Now I'm focused on making my dream real, working during the day and attending classes at night to prepare for auditions. Hey, do you know the most popular question I get asked as an aspiring actress?'

'No, what?'

'Can I have an espresso and a muffin please?'

Joe laughed. 'So, you work in a café?'

'At the moment, yes. But just until I make it!'

'Cool. So do you want to go first and I'll experiment on you?' Joe asked.

'Be my guest,' she replied.

Joe started by watching Caroline's body language as she talked about the things that she was interested in and mismatching her. When she crossed her legs, he opened his. When she leaned toward him, he leaned away. It was a lot of fun and he could see her getting more and more frustrated. As he listened to her speak, he noticed she was talking about the way she *saw* things and about her *focus*, so he started using feeling words back to her: 'I can *feel* this is important to you' and 'I am starting to *grasp* what you're *feeling*.' This made her look even more annoyed. Joe was really enjoying himself.

It took Caroline less than five minutes to totally freak out and exclaim, 'Joe, if you don't stop this right now, I'm going to punch you. Hard!'

Joe couldn't help laughing, but nonetheless apologized. *Wow*, he thought, *she's upset easily.*

Then they moved on to the second part of the exercise. As Joe matched Caroline's body language and representational systems, he found that she smiled more and looked a lot more comfortable in the conversation.

Soon it was time to switch roles and when Joe was on the receiving end of the mismatching, he realized how annoying it was. *Maybe she wasn't being such a whiner, after all*, he admitted to himself.

Caroline could see his growing discomfort and started grinning. 'Ha! Not so nice having the shoe on the other foot, is it? God, this is fun!'

'OK, OK. Now it's your turn to *match* me,' Joe responded quickly.

'Ugh – this is the boring bit,' Caroline said with a smile.

It was a lot of fun to practise matching and mismatching. Joe decided that as soon as he got back home he would put the matching skills he'd just learned into practice with his girlfriend.

Alan soon returned to the stage.

Any questions about the exercise?

He paused and looked at the audience. Seeing that there were no puzzled looks or raised hands, he went on with a smile:

It seems you guys had fun with the whole mismatching business.

Some of the participants looked each other up and down and laughed.

Now, before I move on to the next topic, I'd like to make a short digression that has to do with the techniques and models we're learning. Over the years, a whole lot of techniques have been invented, so today we will only *see* a quick preview and *hear* about the basic concepts to get the *hang* of it. Before everything else, NLP is an attitude, and in this regard, Richard is a true master.

Now it's obviously a good idea for most of your communication that you get along really well with the other person, so rapport-building and using representational systems are of paramount importance. Something else that is vital to becoming an effective communicator is a system known as *the meta model.*

The meta model was one of the first models developed by Richard, along with John Grinder, back in the early days. It came from noticing the way the most successful therapists, like Virginia Satir, asked questions of their clients to help them improve their life.

The meta model has three main functions: to specify information, to clarify information and to help a person open up their model of the world.

On the flipchart in the right-hand corner of the stage Alan wrote:

1. Specify information.
2. Clarify information.
3. Open up a person's model of the world.

By 'model', I mean map of the world. Does this ring any bells?

'The map is not the territory,' Joe heard from across the room.

Exactly. Every time we communicate with others, we are presenting our maps. We are deleting, distorting and generalizing information. Now, sometimes this is useful because it means that we can have conversations that don't last forever. For example, when someone asks you how you are, you can respond that you are well. It's one word, so you're obviously deleting a lot of information, but it serves a purpose.

When we map reality, we delete, generalize and distort the information we receive from our senses. Then, when we describe that map with words – either to others or to ourselves – we do it again: we delete, generalize and distort the map.

When I talk about specifying or clarifying information, what I mean is, to give you an example: you come home from work and your partner tells you there's been an accident. What does this mean? Have they burnt the dinner? Have they broken your favourite vase? Bumped your car? Has someone, heaven forbid, been seriously hurt? Of course you can take a shot in the dark – it happens more often than one would suspect – or you can ask for more details. The meta model helps you ask the right questions, especially when the deletion, generalization and distortion process is less evident. We'll see specifically how later.

Another example would be hearing someone say 'I'm not a people person.'

As Alan looked in his direction, Joe blushed bright red with the realization that he was referring to their conversation earlier that morning.

One good question is: 'What do you mean by "people person"?' Usually, the person will say something like, 'Well, I'm not confident speaking to others.' This already shifts the attention from something they *are* to something they *do* — which is easier to address.

You might continue by asking, 'Is there someone specific you aren't confident speaking to?' With this you allow them to narrow it down and find the specific events behind a widely generalized belief. Now you are one step closer to uncovering the actual territory.

You see, the more you drill down and identify the specific issue, the easier it is for you to help the person find a solution.

Joe couldn't help but start answering the questions that he knew were implicitly meant for him. What had he meant by not being a people person? Was there someone specific he felt unsure about speaking to? What lay behind it?

As he was considering these questions, Alan continued speaking:

The least obvious use of the meta model, and probably the most important, is helping a person enrich their map of the world.

That's what people like Virginia Satir understood and that's what we have modelled from her. What I'm going to give you now is a set of questions that will enable you to do just the same.

But first let's look at an example of how you could expand and enrich somebody's map of the world. If someone says, 'Everybody hates me,' that's a generalization. And it's not likely to be accurate:

the vast majority of the world's population will in fact be unaware of that person's existence and probably wouldn't bother to form an opinion of them if they were aware of it.

So, you can challenge that generalization by questioning the term 'everybody'. When you have got to the bottom of it and found out exactly who they mean, you have already taken a problem that was overwhelming and made it more manageable. You can then work on it even more by asking how they know that this person hates them, what specific episode has brought them to that conclusion, if that episode could be read any other way, and so on. The more you question the belief using the meta model, the more likely you are to sow seeds of doubt in the belief. And that creates room for the person to change that belief to a more useful or resourceful one.

Of course you can begin by questioning your own deletions, generalizations and distortions.

Joe was intrigued: this meta model seemed to be a really powerful tool for communication. It also occurred to him that it would be perfect for changing some of his limiting beliefs.

The closer you can get to the actual sensory experience, the more useful it is. So, as a general rule, try and describe what you saw, what you heard and what you felt. Being specific and sticking to the senses is an excellent way to add details to the map.

Let's talk about some questions that are particularly useful, and I mean in any context. They work in business negotiation, they work when you want to get through to your teenage son or daughter. These are questions that I teach to everyone: people in a relationship, psychologists, senior managers, teachers, salespeople – you name it.

Sometimes you will use these questions to get clarity on what a person is talking about. Say you hired someone to give a stress-management seminar in your company on the assumption that you knew what it might be about. What if the trainer arrived wearing a yellow robe, started lighting scented candles and asked you and your co-workers to get in touch with your animal guides, play the drums and run naked through the corridors? You'd all think him crazy, right?

The audience laughed.

But that's because you never clarified what that particular trainer meant by the term 'stress management'. There is so much confusion and misunderstanding in business, and in life, because people fail to clarify what the other person means. In business it's also important that when you hire someone, you understand specifically what they will do for you, and *how* specifically as well as *when* specifically. These questions allow you to ensure the situation is understood by all parties equally.

Joe smiled to himself. He remembered a number of meetings where big words and acronyms had been thrown about and he had been clueless as to what they meant and spent the entire meeting not understanding what was going on. Later he had discovered that most of the others had had no idea either! He had a feeling this was fairly typical in the corporate world. These meta-model questions would provide him with a real opportunity to understand his colleagues more easily.

Alan was moving on:

> I can see some of you beginning to pay more attention to the empty flipchart than to what I'm saying, so let's proceed.

And with that he turned to a new flipchart page and wrote:

HOW? WHAT? WHEN? WHERE? WHO SPECIFICALLY?

These questions not only help you to get past a person's generalizations and drill down to what they are actually talking about, they also help you to get more information about exactly what they are doing inside their head. For example, when someone says, 'I'm just finding it all a struggle at the moment,' you can ask, 'Finding what exactly a struggle?' or 'How specifically are you finding it a struggle?' This allows them to define for you the exact problem and how it is a problem for them. This cuts through to the core of the issue very quickly. You can use these specific questions to get a real understanding of what's going on.

WHO SAYS? ACCORDING TO WHOM?

This question, however you phrase it, is a powerful way of turning what is stated as a fact into an opinion. Often when people give voice to their beliefs, they will word them as if they were true statements. When you ask, 'Who says?' the answer they give repositions the statement as an opinion rather than a fact. Of course, an opinion is just an opinion and isn't necessarily true. For example, if someone says, 'People don't like me,' and you ask this question, then they will have to own the belief. More than likely the sentence will become 'I believe that people don't like me.' The moment you phrase it as an opinion, you make it easier for change to happen.

This made a lot of sense to Joe. He had to admit he often made statements as if they were absolutely true when they were really just what he was feeling at the time. Even that thing about being a people person fell into this category!

Alan continued writing on the chart:

EVERYBODY? ALWAYS? NEVER? NOBODY? NOTHING? ALL? NO ONE?

Another category that we've seen in the example that I gave you before and that you will encounter is that of over-generalization. Listen for words such as 'always', 'never' and 'everybody'. When you hear those words, you can challenge the statement simply by repeating the word. 'Always?' 'Everybody?' 'Never?'

WHAT DO YOU MEAN BY THAT?

As well as this question being incredibly useful to clarify what a person is thinking, it can also be used to challenge a person's belief when they speak about more abstract concepts. For example, often people will talk about the fact that they 'have' depression or that panic 'follows' them everywhere. Distortions like this are very common, because people feel that this is what is happening. When you ask them to clarify what they mean, usually they will restate the problem in more process-oriented terms – they might say that they 'feel' depressed or that they 'panic'. If they present the problem as something they do, then they have the ability to do something different instead.

COMPARED TO WHOM? COMPARED TO WHAT?

One of the things that people often do to limit themselves is to evaluate themselves in relation to others. They say things like 'I'm no good at this' and when you ask the question 'Compared to whom?' it forces them to see that they are making an unfair comparison that isn't useful. If you feel bad because you feel you aren't good at golf and I ask you, 'Compared to whom?' you'll more than likely compare yourself to someone professional. Once you have to identify this, it's easier for you to understand that it is, in fact, an unfair comparison.

Many female friends of mine, for example, compare themselves to the prettiest and slimmest models they see in magazines or the most beautiful girls they walk past in the city, and that makes them feel bad.

As human beings, we often focus on our flaws and compare ourselves in those areas to others. Low self-esteem is the result of feeling bad compared to other people. By challenging such comparisons, we get to realize that we all have good points and bad points, and because we are all unique, the only valid comparison we can actually make is when we compare ourselves now to ourselves in the past. That way we don't have to feel bad about who we are.

This really rang true for Joe. In the past he had continuously told himself that he was no good and wasn't smart and, although he no longer said those things very often, he still felt bad in some social situations. As he dwelt on this issue, he realized he was still continuously comparing himself to those around him.

HOW DO YOU KNOW?

One of the most damaging beliefs is when people convince themselves that they know what another person is thinking or what will happen in the future. They might think that someone doesn't like them or that something isn't going to work out for them, and that can cause them a lot of problems.

A great question you can use to challenge such beliefs is: 'How do you know?' This forces them to explain how they reached that conclusion. When they try and do so, often it will become apparent that they are basing their belief on faulty assumptions.

So, for example, imagine you believe that someone doesn't like you and I ask you, 'How do you know?' The answer you might give is that they didn't say hello to you at a party. However, there may have been a number of reasons why they didn't say hello. This effectively challenges your conclusion.

I might ask you, 'So every time someone doesn't say hello to you at a party, it's because they don't like you?'

Notice that I'm using a generalization – 'every time' – so, if you actually answered, 'Yes,' how would I challenge you?

'Every time?' someone in the audience asked.

Exactly! It looks as if you're getting the hang of it. Excellent.

Another example might be if you were to say to me that you'd never pass your driving test. Again, if I were to ask you, 'How do you know?' at best you'd point to what had happened in the past as evidence for what would happen in the future. Of course, the past doesn't equal the future, so again your belief would be challenged.

'How do you know?' forces a person to examine the logic they have used in coming to their conclusion and enables you to highlight the flaws inherent in such logic.

WHAT STOPS YOU? WHAT WOULD HAPPEN IF YOU COULD?

When you hear someone say 'I can't ...' or 'I'm not able to ...', these two questions allow you to challenge those limits.

The question 'What stops you?' helps you figure out what obstacles lie between where you are now and where you want to be. It enables you to identify the challenges that you think you'll have to face in order to get what you want. Once those challenges become clear, knowing what to do will be easier. Sometimes they will be about resources or some specific knowledge you need to acquire, while other times they will be about beliefs you might have to change in order to succeed.

The question 'What would happen if you could?' gets you to imagine yourself overcoming all the obstacles and achieving the result. This gives you the sense that it is, in fact, possible. Used in conjunction, these questions are really powerful.

For example, I worked with a teacher who told me that she couldn't get through to her students. When I asked her, 'What stops you?' she told me that they didn't listen to her, she didn't have their respect and they had their phones on in class. I asked her if sorting out those three issues would ensure that she could get through to her students and she agreed that it would. So then she had three things she knew she could do. To help even more, I asked her, 'What would happen if you could get through to your students?' She immediately sat up and explained how happy she would be and that she would see them improving and enjoying the lessons. It made a remarkable difference to her attitude towards something that had her feel powerless for quite some time.

WHAT WOULD HAPPEN IF YOU DID? WHAT WOULD HAPPEN IF YOU DIDN'T?

Lastly, when decisions need to be made, these two questions can help hugely by opening up a world of possible outcomes. When someone thinks they must or should do something, they're usually held back by beliefs about what would or wouldn't happen if they did or didn't do that thing. Get those beliefs out in the open, because most of the time they are the real issue and challenging them will help the person to make the best decision.

For example, I had a client who felt that she 'had to' keep the same job even though she hated it. I asked her those questions and she allowed herself to explore parts of her map that, while remaining out of her awareness, had nonetheless been putting a lot of pressure on her. She was then able to review her options with greater understanding and new peace of mind, and she found it easier to discover something she actually did enjoy.

Joe gazed up at the flipchart. This stuff really made sense. He was transfixed. There were so many questions that he could be using to improve both his thinking and his communication. He put a big exclamation mark beside the questions he had copied down in his journal.

Alan continued:

The questions I have written down are just some of those you can use to specify and clarify information as well as help people change their beliefs and perceptions and open up their model of the world. And, as you will have noticed, they are all very simple, very conversational. It's not about asking fancy questions that no one would understand anyway, it's about posing the right question at the right moment. And that skill, of course, requires practice, so – time to try it out for yourselves!

What I want you to do now is to get into pairs and each of you in turn to work on an issue the other person has. When you use these questions, you will find yourself getting to the heart of the matter very quickly and it will help them change the way they think about things.

One word of advice: these questions are very personal and very direct. Remember always to establish and maintain rapport, otherwise the only answer you'll get is a horrible look. Is that understood?

OK. Now go and do the exercise, and be nice to each other. Richard will see you here in 30 minutes and he will share with you his personal insights on language.

Joe and Emily glanced at each other and decided to work together.

'OK! So, how can I help you today, Emily?' Joe began with a grin.

Emily hesitated for a long time before answering, 'There's something I feel bad about and I don't know what to do about it. I can't tell anybody, but it's ruining my life.'

This sounded serious! Joe didn't know where to begin. He wondered how this issue could be ruining Emily's whole life. He decided to use a question that challenged her generalization: 'What do you mean by "ruining your life"? Is every part of your life connected to this problem? Is your whole life doomed as a result? Is it going to affect your health as well?'

'No ... I mean, it's just really difficult for me. I can't tell anyone.'

'Well, what would happen if you could change things?'

Emily considered the question. 'Well, I suppose I would ... I would feel better ... and things would be OK.'

Joe wanted to ask *what* the problem was, but he realized that Emily wasn't in a good state and that he needed to build more rapport with her and make her feel more comfortable first. So, he began to pace her breathing and then, in a softer tone, he matched the auditory terms that she had used.

'It's OK, Emily. If you decide not to tell me anything, that's fine. But I might just try a few more questions if that's OK? You never know. I might be able to help.'

Emily smiled, feeling somewhat more at ease. 'OK, Joe. Although I'm not sure how it could make that much of a difference. We might as well go for it, though, and see where it takes us.'

Joe noticed this time she had used the word 'see' and decided to match her visual preference.

'Great. OK, then. Let's see if together we can get a new perspective on this problem. What stops you from telling people, Emily?'

Emily paused. She frowned and held her breath. 'I feel I will have let them down.'

Joe noticed that she was being vague and hadn't specified who 'they' were. He wanted to get more clarity.

'You feel that you would let them down? Let whom down specifically?'

Emily looked over at Teresa, then looked back at Joe.

Joe picked up on it. 'Is it Teresa, Emily? Are you afraid to tell your mum?'

Emily looked at him nervously and nodded slowly.

Joe realized that Emily felt that she already knew how Teresa would react. He decided to challenge this assumption.

'How do you know Teresa will feel let down, Emily?'

'I just ... well, I'm just worried ...'

'You're worried. Do you think your mother loves you, Emily?'

Emily nodded.

'Do you really think she's going to feel let down by you or do you think that maybe she might understand?'

'I don't want to disappoint her. If she realizes that I ... well, that I can't stand up for myself ... There's this bully at school and she ... she makes my life hell.'

Emily started welling up as she looked intently at Joe, waiting for his reaction.

Joe paused for a moment, unsure how to take it from here. He wanted to help Emily see that there were more options and that her mother could be part of the solution, not the problem. He remembered a question that might just help: 'What would happen if you gave your mum the possibility of knowing that her daughter needed her help?'

As he spoke, it dawned on Joe that the problem that Emily was having was very similar to the one that Teresa had told him about earlier. It seemed to him that mother and daughter were struggling with a similar issue. While Emily was getting bullied, Teresa found it difficult to deal with aggressive people.

Joe felt sure the meta-model questions were really helping Emily sort things out, but he wasn't finished yet. There was one more thing he wanted to explore.

'Emily, you said this bully made your life hell. What do you mean by that?'

Emily paused and then said, 'Well, she teases me in front of everyone else and she shouts at me and calls me names. I'm stupid.'

It occurred to Joe that Emily wasn't getting her information from a reliable source.

'Who says?' he enquired.

'The bully,' she responded.

'Stupid compared to whom, Emily? Compared to the bully?'

A small smile appeared on Emily's face. 'Well, no. Actually, the bully is way stupider than I am.' She giggled.

Joe smiled back at her. 'So, are you really stupid if she's the one saying it?'

Emily looked up and shook her head.

'Next time that bully comes along,' Joe continued, 'you feel sorry for her. She's probably attacking you because she feels stupid herself.'

By the end of their talk, Emily felt a lot better about her problem and had decided it was time for her to open up to her mother about what was going on. She wiped her eyes and smiled at Joe. It looked as though a weight had been lifted from her shoulders.

For his part, Joe felt elated about how powerful some questions could be in helping a person see things from a different perspective. He decided to spend some time studying the Meta Model and understanding how he could apply it in his personal and professional life.

Next it was time for Emily to practise the meta-model questions on Joe.

'So, Joe, I might take a bit of time as I question you, if that's OK? We have an old proverb that goes: *if you don't know the way, walk slowly.*'

Joe smiled as he nodded, imagining Emily with a pint of Guinness in front of her.

'So, anyway, what's going on for you then, Joe?'

He sighed. It was time for him to talk about what had really been troubling him.

'I'm a disaster when it comes to being a good boyfriend.'

'What do you mean by "disaster"?' Emily asked.

'Well, because I drive her mad.'

'Always?' Emily continued.

'Not always, no.'

'Uh, let's see,' Emily said, looking at the flipchart. 'How do you drive her mad, specifically?'

'I – well, I don't know. When she's upset I always say the wrong thing.'

'Aha – *a closed mouth, a wise head.*'

'What?'

'Oh, never mind. I'm just joking,' Emily continued. 'So, you say the wrong thing *every* time?'

'Well, no … but sometimes I just can't seem to say the right thing!'

'What stops you from doing that?'

'I don't know. I do seem to spend a lot of time asking her if it's anything to do with me.'

Joe paused for a few seconds and thought about what he just said. This was a big insight for him. He realized that he actually made things worse by asking that question and focusing on himself.

Emily continued, 'Joe, what would happen if, instead of asking if it had to do with you, you focused on what she needed at that moment?'

'In that case, I guess I would actually be of help to her.'

'How specifically can you do that in the future?'

Joe paused for a moment. 'You know, there are a lot of things I could do to make her feel good. I feel so much better about it now. You really are your mother's daughter, aren't you? That was amazing, Emily.'

Emily blushed and smiled brightly.

At that moment, Richard returned to the stage and thanked Alan.

While you were practising meta modelling each other, I was sneaking around the room and hearing some great examples.

You know, people don't always ask the most useful questions. For example, if someone comes in and goes, 'I'm depressed,' they often ask, 'About what?' People who train with me don't ask that question, and do you know why? Because we don't want to know the answer. We don't care what they're depressed about and we don't care how they depress themselves. It's not because we're unsympathetic, but because that would just allow us to discover a strategy for how to depress other people about the same thing in the same way – and we have a whole other goal in mind.

I always say to these people, 'How do you know you're depressed? Maybe you're not.'

They always look at me and go, 'Well, I'm pretty sure I'm depressed.'

'Are you depressed while you're sleeping?'

'Gee ... I don't know.'

Then I explain, 'Well, then you're probably not. Now, are there other times when you're not depressed?'

And typically they look back and go, 'Well, there was this time when I was happy, but when I think about it now ... I don't know.'

Which means that they can distort anything in the past. The problem is that they do the same thing when they look into the future. My policy is simple: the best thing about the past is that it's over.

HOW TO BECOME A MASTERFUL COMMUNICATOR

To me it's not just your problem that's a problem — it's the actual way you think about it.

Virginia never asked people why they were shy. She asked what would happen if they weren't. Because, you see, asking why just keeps people in their own map, which is the reason why they're screwed up in the first place. Instead, a question like 'What would happen if you weren't?' takes a person to the edge of their map and opens it up to new possibilities.

Virginia and Milton believed that everybody could change. They never gave up, just as I don't. The thing is that people have all kinds of beliefs, and these beliefs are as strong and real as anything else. That's what stops people from being able to act in new ways. The bottom line is this: if you believe strongly enough that a person can change, then you can make that person join you in that belief, and they will actually make it happen.

Now, a quick word about language. There are examples of language misuse all over the country. I saw a place the other day with a sign on the outside that said: 'Centre for Sexual Dysfunction.' I drive around in the United States and I think, *These guys know nothing about how language works*. 'One-Hour Pain Clinic.' I thought there was enough of that going around already.

I get business cards from people that say they're 'alcoholic counsellors' or 'medical specialists for chronic pain' and I don't think you need to be a specialist for that. There's enough pain in the world as it is. I think you need to be a specialist in making people feel good and in gaining control. Because, after all, if you can have a paper cut and it doesn't hurt until you see it, then there are some things that aren't worth looking at.

And one word I hate? 'Disabled.' I don't know about you guys, but I find it really aggravating. To me, the people who are born with a brain that doesn't learn the same way other people's brains learn aren't disabled. They're inconvenienced, because what we have is not a learning disability but a teaching disability. I know I gave psychologists a hard time. I know I gave teachers a hard time as well, but, you see, it's not their fault. It's not teachers' fault that they've never been taught the best way to teach children. They go to school, but nobody teaches them anything about how to teach. So, people aren't handicapped; they're only inconvenienced. And they're inconvenienced only because we have structured the world in a certain way.

The only loose end that you need to tie up now is to stop and realize that what you have learned in this workshop is to trust yourself. If you go into the right state, the answers about how to do things will come to you.

You just really have to listen to people. People don't just talk metaphorically. If you really listen to them, they'll tell you exactly what you need to know.

But if you ask questions such as 'Why are you screwed up?', they'll give you reasons, and that's not going to help them to see outside their box. The beauty of the meta model is that it gives you a roadmap to navigate your way beyond what is known territory.

Now when you leave here, there's something that's going to happen to you. You're going to start to hear things that have been there all along. People are going to start to say things to you like, 'Well, you know, I just keep telling myself this isn't going to work, and it makes me pessimistic.' And you're going to look at them and say, 'Now, take the voice that tells you it's not going to work and make it sound untrustworthy.' Or get them to challenge what it says through the questions of the meta model.

This is about figuring out how to get where you want to go and, more importantly, wanting to go somewhere worth going.

I don't want you to repeat my 40 years of history so that you almost get to where I've got to, I want you to jump to the end and go on. That makes a lot more sense to me. And if you've been worrying or feeling anxious, I want you to start finding your worries hilarious.

Liz, where are you?

Liz put up her hand.

I want you thinking about all your problems. Think about them now.

The audience went silent and everyone turned to Liz, who burst out laughing.

You see, it's not merely something that makes you feel better just in the moment – the changes last. Food for thought. Now let's have a short break and I'll meet you back here in 20 minutes for the last part of this seminar.

Joe went for a walk outside, relishing the chance to process what he had been learning. There were a lot of things to think about and Joe knew that it was really important to apply what he was learning in the real world.

Later, on the way back into the seminar room, he bumped into Liz. 'Well done on getting up there,' he said.

'Thanks.' Liz smiled. 'It's amazing how much more relaxed I feel. I can't wait to get back home and back to the classroom and start doing some serious rethinking.'

Joe laughed.

Liz continued, 'How have you been enjoying the workshop?'

'Terrific. Richard is a riot, and this meta-model stuff – it's fascinating how powerful language can be.'

They chatted their way to the coffee table and Joe noted that Liz really did look much more relaxed than she had that morning.

'It's crazy how dramatic the change can be, isn't it?' he observed.

Liz nodded. 'Yes. To be honest, I couldn't believe it myself. I mean, I get stressed out really quickly, but when I started to spin the feelings, I started to just feel lighter. Do you know what I mean?'

Joe nodded encouragingly.

'And even having just done it once gives me confidence that I can turn other things around as well. I know I have it in me and if I think about the things that used to stress me out, now I just …' Liz started giggling and immediately Joe started feeling lighter too. He was delighted.

After chatting to Liz for a few more minutes, he went back to his seat. The music started and Richard appeared onstage.

Chapter 5

HOW TO CREATE A WONDERFUL LIFE

Usually a person's problem isn't the most important problem. The biggest problem is that they spend so much time on it that if they do get rid of it, they just start filling their time up with new crap. Instead, I like them to look into the future and have it full of wonderful feelings.

Over the years, I've had to do all kinds of things to convince people not to accept limitations. Constantly, I've had to demonstrate things. You see, it's not by putting up a fight that you solve your problems. If you're planning to quit smoking, the worst thing you can do is try to resist the urge. You say to yourself, 'Don't smoke cigarettes. Don't want cigarettes. Don't think about cigarettes.' But that way, all you ever think about is cigarettes, cigarettes, cigarettes!

When you tell someone *not* to think about something, their brain must first picture the thing you told them not to think of and then negate it. The problem is that at this point they're already heading in the wrong direction.

What you do instead is notice the sensations of craving. Then you turn them up and point the feeling in the right direction. I have worked with people who were literally dying from eating too much chocolate – their liver was shutting down because of all the chocolate. So I put chocolate on a chair and I had them look at the chair and realize that the chocolate had more willpower than they had. 'Look at it,' I said. 'It's smarter than you are, it's got more tenacity than you have and it's got control over its behaviour. It can keep its wrapper on. You can't.'

'Well,' they'd answer, 'I feel stupid.'

'But not stupid enough.'

'What?'

'Take that feeling of stupidity now and start to turn it up, because the more you take the feeling of being stupid and the more you spin it around, the sooner you'll reach a point where it's ridiculous. Then, when you look at it, you'll start laughing. It's not through fighting your desires that you're going to become smarter, it's through taking those desires and aiming them where you really need them. Because it's not the desire that's bad, it's the fact that it's pointing to chocolate.

When you take that same feeling of desire and point it to your future, and you desire better health, and you desire more success, and you desire being nicer to the people around you, *then* you will make progress. Because if you vibrate all kinds of things like happiness, like joy, like excitement, then, as I've said, people around you will start doing it too without even knowing what happened.

This was a big realization for Joe. He had been trying so hard to *stop* feeling shy around people. He had also focused a lot on *not* being frustrated with his girlfriend. Instead he decided that he was going to focus on how confident and fun he wanted to be and on what he loved about her. It was just a switch in the other direction, but he was confident it was going to make a significant difference.

Richard continued:

Now, to me, it's not enough that you overcome your problems. I want you to find a way to replace them with new behaviours and new thoughts that take you in a new direction. I want to see you build an incredibly wonderful future and design all kinds of good feelings in it.

And to begin with, I want a volunteer. Who wants to feel really good without a specific reason for the rest of their life?

A number of hands went up. Richard picked Caroline, the actress Joe had worked with earlier. She went onstage and sat down. Once he had found out her name, Richard said:

Caroline, so you would like to feel ridiculously good, yes?

Caroline nodded and smiled.

To do that, you have to tell me something. When you think about the future, where are the images located? When you think of next year, where do you see the images? Are they in front of you? To your left or right? Behind you?

And when you think about the past, where are the images located? Think of a year ago, for instance. Where do you see that image?

After a moment or so, Caroline pointed her right hand out in front of her and gestured behind her with her left hand. 'The future seems to be in front out there and the past is behind me.'

OK. Now, that's one particular way of sorting time in your mind.

If you draw an imaginary line from your past to your future, that would be called your *timeline*.

Having the past in front of you to the left means that it's easier for you to access it. Having it behind you means it's easier for you to forget it. So, for example, you want the lessons you learned in front of you and the negative feelings behind you.

Joe had never thought about how he saw the future and the past before. He began to concentrate and found out that he sorted his future in front of him, a little to the right, while his past ran sideways, to his left.

Richard continued:

The way you sort time determines how you feel about it. What I'm interested in you doing now, Caroline, is learning to build intense feelings of bliss in your future so that you can feel wonderful about your past as well.

Before we get there, is there anything in particular that has bothered you and stopped you from doing what you really want to do?

Caroline nodded. 'Well, I'm a budding actress and I've started doing auditions lately. It's just that I feel really disappointed when I don't get the part that I apply for.'

OK, the first thing is that disappointment requires adequate planning. You have to plan ahead of time in order to feel disappointed. So, how would you like to feel instead of bad? I mean, you want to be able to feel determined, motivated and passionate when you think about an audition, right?

'Yes. I'd like to feel optimistic about the future, and when I think about an audition, I'd love to feel confident that I have a real chance of getting the part and that I deserve to succeed.'

Good move. Wouldn't it be fantastic if you could find a way to change how you felt about the negative experiences in the past and simultaneously develop a belief in a better future?

'Absolutely,' she responded enthusiastically. 'That would be amazing. I just seem to focus on the rejections too much.'

For one thing, I believe that people take rejection too personally. I mean, when someone rejects you, it's not because they planned specifically on being mean to you. It's really just information about the fact that there is either something you are not doing yet or something that you are doing and should stop doing. And either way, the best response is determination and flexibility.

So, Caroline, here's what I want you to do. I want you to just allow your breathing to slow down and to let yourself go effortlessly into a state of comfort. I want you to soften your body and let yourself feel as relaxed as you possibly can. Every breath helps you feel more and more relaxed. Let your eyes close … now.

Richard began to speak more slowly and his voice became even more resonant as he continued:

As you drift all the way into comfort and softness, I want you to begin to imagine yourself drifting up above your timeline and looking down on your past, present and future.

Now I know that as you look down at the past, you can see all those times you went for an audition and didn't get the part. And as you look down at those experiences from this perspective, you can realize that each of those experiences was a training ground for your future success. So what I want you to do is to notice what useful information emerges from each of those experiences. Let it float out above your timeline as a radiant glow. Take that light with you and leave the rest behind, in the past, where it belongs.

Then I want you to put together the best feeling you can imagine. Think of a time when you were feeling on top of the world, when you felt happier than ever. Can you think of a time where you felt really, really good?

With her eyes closed, looking very relaxed, Caroline nodded slowly and smiled.

Make sure you're reliving that experience, now. And as you focus on that wonderful sensation, really begin to build it up and intensify it. Imagine it moving through your body. Now I want you to imagine taking this feeling, giving it the colour that suits you best and spraying it all the way through your past so that it covers every negative memory, every bad time, soaking them in this really great feeling.

I want you to imagine looking down and seeing how your past looks so different now, and feeling so good about all those experiences, and realizing that whatever troubled you is now behind you and getting farther away by the second.

Caroline grinned hugely.

Because the truth is, Caroline, some things are worth forgetting and some things are worth remembering. Many people settle, but what I want you to do, as you feel good about your past, is to imagine looking down at your future and imagine the best kinds of feelings raining down on it, filling every future experience with the best states.

I want you to see your future looking better than ever before, brighter than ever before, more compelling than ever before.

It's time for you to float back into your body, Caroline, so that you can feel full of excitement and anticipation for the most amazing future full of the most wonderful things – new people, new opportunities, new possibilities ... a world of possibilities. Imagine going into the next audition, and the next, with determination, excitement, passion and self-belief.

And slowly you can start to come all the way back, feeling wonderfully good.

Richard paused and Caroline slowly but surely became more aware and opened her eyes, an extremely bright smile on her face.

I guess we don't really need to ask, but ... how do you feel?

Caroline took a deep breath. 'As if I was awake for the first time in months. Everything kind of looks different. I'm going to take Hollywood by storm!'

Richard turned to the audience:

Now, if you auditioned a woman radiating this kind of energy, wouldn't you just beg her to take part in your movie? Of course you would. That's what I mean when I tell you that you need to get into the right state, whatever it is that you're about to do.

Let's give Caroline a round of applause.

Caroline bounced off the stage and back to her chair.

And now, for those of you who actually thought I was doing this just for Caroline …

Richard looked down at the audience.

Let yourself relax and let your eyes close. At this time of day, if you begin to look at things as if they're difficult, they will be; if you begin to study what makes things impossible, you'll find out. And if somebody comes in with a problem, they can get rid of it, but that's not the most important thing. The most important thing is this: when you get rid of that problem, what are you going to do with all of the spare time that you'll have?

People really need to learn to orient themselves toward a brighter future. And that begins by learning how to feel really good. So the first thing I want you to do is practise. Now, take a deep breath and just let your consciousness float comfortably with every deep breath you take … in through your nose and out through your mouth …

Now, if you're talking to yourself inside your head, I don't care what you're saying, as long as you slow the voice down. And soften it.

And as you soften it, just remember to keep breathing, because I want you to learn to adjust your state. And if your consciousness goes to a place that feels tight, then go to a place in your body where you feel totally relaxed. Let the relaxation spread. The rest will take care of itself.

Now, think of something absolutely wonderful from your own life. See what you saw at that time, hear what you heard and get back some wonderful sensations. In fact, let's see if we can take the five best experiences in your life and make them the foundation for your future. Lots of people go into their past and pick all the crappy things that happened to them and then think about what will happen in the future. Instead, I'd like you, from this relaxed state, to simply go back and find five wonderful things – things that made you feel special, times when you surprised yourself delightfully – and then connect these things together. Think of the first one, the second one, the third one, the fourth one, the fifth one, and cycle back to the beginning. And remember to step inside these good experiences. See what you saw when you were there. Let them run through your mind.

Ask yourself, 'What does it feel like to be in a state of bliss?' Because in order to answer that question, you have to go into a state of bliss, and the more you do it, the better you become at mastering how to feel good for no reason whatsoever, other than you're alive and you deserve it.

And when you've run through those five experiences, look into the future and add a sixth one. Think about something you're going to do when you leave this workshop, something you're going to do differently.

Train your neurology to go through the best of who you are and the best of what you've done, and then think about what you're going to do about this stuff. This is the new you, and the truth is that you can learn new things, and so can the people around you. You can meet people and instead of feeling frustrated, you can keep smiling, and when you get into this state, suddenly they're going to go into the same state, because yoghurt knows yoghurt, and bliss knows bliss. And optimism and hope are what people need, no matter who they are, whether an employee, somebody you're trying to sell a car to, or the people you love the most.

You want to make it so that your optimism always prevails. The only time you ever lose is when you stop. So stopping isn't the activity you want. You want to build more tenacity.

Now the trick is not to come out of this state but to go through it so that when you come out the other side, you don't feel the same anymore. You don't want to go back to who you were; you want to go on to who you can be.

You begin with your thoughts, then thoughts become actions, actions become habits, and habits become part of who you truly are. So, now it's time to turn new thoughts into new behaviour, into trying new things. You find yourself doing things you enjoy, you find yourself being kinder to people and you find yourself being more patient. And it's time to realize that all the suffering you've been doing – you've done it beautifully. And now that you've mastered that, it's time to discover the answer to the question 'How much pleasure can you stand?'

So tonight, while you sleep and dream, I want all of those bad habits, all of those bad nightmares, all of those bad repetitive things you did – the self-criticism, the low self-esteem, the worrying about meeting people, the shyness, whether it's emotional or physical – to stop.

For many people it's spiritual, because in the societies in which we live, we have chopped off all kinds of important things about our own spirit. So, if you have ever been told you'd never amount to anything, if you have ever been told you were stupid, if you have ever been told anything like that, I want you to hear a mantra inside your head that says, 'Screw that!' Because it's simply not true.

I've seen thousands and thousands of people change in thousands and thousands of ways, even when I was told it was impossible. And if you think you're impervious to good feelings, just wait until you're sleeping, because when all these other things come back to your mind, I want your unconscious to give you an unexplainable sense of well-being. In fact, there's no better time to start than now, as you sit here. I know your unconscious can hear, so it doesn't matter when you do it, as long as your unconscious responds fully and you start to allow a smile to creep across your face and down throughout your body. Because it's time for you to slowly but surely come all the way back to full consciousness, bringing a warm glow with you, a sense of delight and a big bright smile.

Joe slowly came to and felt himself smiling all the way through his body. He felt fantastic.

Richard thanked Alan and the other assistants and went on to say:

Today you've been exposed to a vast number of ideas and some you'll remember right away and some will come up and surprise you along the way. Yet there's one thing that I expect you to know when you leave here: I expect you to know that if you are doing something and it's not working, there's got to be an easier way.

And if whatever you're doing isn't working, then you've got to do something else. And the first thing you've got to do is change your own internal state. Because if you feel frustrated, people around you will pick up on that and you'll just get stuck.

Relax and people will relax too. Feel good and things will get better!

A standing ovation later, Richard left the stage. As he did so, Joe turned to Teresa and Emily and suggested a trip to the local coffee shop before they said their goodbyes. They agreed and invited Edgar as well.

As Joe was making his way towards the door, he heard his name called. It was Alan.

'Well?' he asked.

Joe nodded. 'Yes, it was ... It's made a difference to me.'

Alan smiled. 'You know, Joe, what we talked about earlier? I really hope you're going to apply what you've learned here to your life, especially your love life. Years ago, I let an incredible woman slip through my fingers because I made a lot of mistakes. I've moved on from there, but still, when I see someone like you who has found a great girl, I want to make sure *you* make the most of it.'

Joe nodded. This came as a bit of a surprise to him, but it explained Alan's intensity earlier.

'Thanks so much for everything.'

'Happy to help, Joe. I hope I get to see you again. And good luck with everything.'

Joe embraced Alan and said his goodbyes.

He soon caught up with the others, who had been joined by a few more participants from the course, including Caroline.

Minutes later, Joe found himself in a coffee shop having a great time chatting about the course. He looked at the assembled company and noticed that they all had very similar postures and were matching each other. He smiled to himself.

Turning his attention to Edgar, he asked him what he had thought of the seminar.

'It was very good,' Edgar replied. 'I certainly got what I was looking for. I mean, what we learned here doesn't really make much of a difference unless we apply it, but I've definitely got some new skills I'm going to use. That state-changing stuff we did where we learned to white out bad memories and spin and anchor in good feelings was amazing. It adds to all the stuff I got before.' Edgar returned to his squeaky Yoda voice. 'A fun and useful experience it was. Happy am I.'

'Yes,' Joe grinned, shaking his head. 'Funny you are! I do know what you mean, though. It just shows what's possible.'

'And the meta-model questions are going to be particularly handy for me. I already use lots of them, but now I can do so even more deliberately.'

Joe thought back to the various tools and skills he had acquired during the course. He agreed with Edgar. What he liked about NLP was that it was full of practical skills, not just a lot of hype and positive thinking. He would set his mind to the task of applying it immediately.

Teresa interrupted his thoughts. 'Joe, Emily has just opened up to me about what has been going on with her. Thank you so much for the work you did with her.'

'Not at all, Teresa. She helped me a lot as well, you know.'

'I've no doubt about that. It's funny, isn't it, that both of us have been letting bullies intimidate us. Well, no more. From now on my daughter and I are going to stand up for ourselves. We've made a pact.'

A huge smile crossed Joe's face.

'Joe,' Teresa continued, 'please send my regards and best thoughts to the love of your life. She will probably grill you on what you've learned.'

Joe nodded and Edgar chimed in, 'If you want my advice, Joe, when she asks about the course, just tell her you don't remember anything because you spent the whole seminar thinking of her!'

Teresa and Joe both laughed. 'Thanks for the advice, Edgar. Smooth. Very smooth.'

Emily joined the chat. 'So, Joe, what's next?'

'Well, next I plan to go home and spend more time getting to know my beautiful girlfriend and then to get on much better with people at my workplace. I really feel I have the ...'

Joe was interrupted by Emily pretending to sleep and snore.

'Ha, ha, ha! Very funny!' Joe exclaimed.

Teresa and Edgar giggled.

'You know, another thing I got from this seminar,' Joe said, 'was the importance of humour. I mean, it was a consistent underlying message about how to become free and happy. Problems are worth laughing at. Life is worth laughing at. Laughter makes it easier to change things. When we can laugh at ourselves, our issues and our worlds, then we can really be free.'

Everyone nodded. Joe had the feeling he had made a few more friends he would be staying in touch with.

After spending some more time chatting, Joe heard his phone ring. He looked at the caller ID, smiled and excused himself. As he walked outside, a strong feeling of excitement moved through his body. Noticing this, he immediately anchored it. Then he answered the phone. It was time to start using what he had learned.

Chapter 6

AFTER THE WORKSHOP

A month later, Joe arrived home from work one evening feeling happy and excited. He had really improved his relationship with some of his colleagues and had found himself understanding them a lot more. Just the night before, when they had all gone out for drinks after a presentation at the office, he had had the unexpected and welcome feeling that a few of them even looked up to him.

After he had made himself a cup of tea and sat down on the couch, he picked up his journal from the coffee table. He started reading through it, proud that he had implemented many of the skills and concepts he had learned only a few weeks before. From a work perspective, he had really made an effort and was reaping the rewards, including popularity, as a result. Of course, he still had to be careful and was fully aware that he would face challenges ahead, but he was content that he was getting better at figuring out the needs and desires of others, be they his colleagues, his superiors or his customers.

As Joe flicked through the pages of his journal, his thoughts moved to his girlfriend. This was the big day: the day that she was due to move in. Joe had applied many of the rapport skills that he learned to his communication with his girlfriend as well and found they were getting on much better as a result. Still, he knew that they were both on a high because she was moving in and the real challenge was to come.

Just then the door opened and his girlfriend walked in.

Joe's immediate excitement at seeing her was tempered when he saw her face. Her eyes were red and she was crying. Joe stood up, unsure of what to do, as she made her way to the nearest chair and slumped into it. Straightaway, he started to think the worst. Frozen to the spot, he looked at her, searching for a sign that she had decided she didn't want to move in, or, worse, to be with him anymore. He didn't know what to think as she just curled over, put her head in her hands and sobbed. Every part of him wanted to ask her if it was about him, if she didn't love him anymore, if she wanted to leave him.

But then he remembered what he had learned. For the first time in such a situation, he asked himself, *How do you know it's about you, Joe? Is everything in her life about you? Of course not. What does she need right now?*

Marching straight over to her and putting his arms around her, he whispered in her ear, 'I'm so sorry you're upset, princess, but whatever it is we'll get through it.'

Without warning, she grabbed him, held him tight and nestled her head into his shoulder. Through the tears, she started speaking.

'Sorry, Joe. It's just been a horrible day with the book. I've lost my creativity.'

'What do you mean?' Joe asked softly.

'Well, I showed my agent a proposal for a new book and she hated it. She looked bored with it. Bored with me.'

That's it? Joe thought to himself. *That's no reason to be so upset.*

Fortunately, for the second time that evening, he had the sense to think twice before opening his mouth.

This isn't about what you think. This is about her map of the world. To her it is a big deal.

'Listen,' he said, 'I know it looks bad at the moment, but I'm very sure your agent decided to be your agent because she saw how much talent you had and viewed you as a really important author.'

His girlfriend looked up at him, wiping her eyes. 'You really think so?'

Joe nodded with a smile. 'I know so. You are incredible at what you do. Your first book was really good, you got an amazing publishing deal and you are so creative I know you'll come up with a terrific idea for another book very soon. It's just about seeing what you can do to look for more ideas that might work.'

Slowly, she nodded. She was no longer crying.

Joe continued, 'Besides, remember, today is the most important day of your life: today you move in with the most handsome man in the world.'

She giggled. 'But I thought I was moving in with you!'

Joe grabbed her and started tickling her, and they exploded into laughter.

Chapter 7

JOE'S JOURNAL

Notes from the Workshop

- 'You're never done learning.' If you feel you know everything there is to know, you're obviously missing something!

- The map is not the territory: your understanding of the world is based on how you represent it (your map), not on the world itself.

- Whatever you think is going on, remember that it's just a map.

- Trouble begins when your map doesn't match the maps of the people around you.

119

- To have better options, better feelings and better interactions with others, you need to expand your map. You need to be able to look at the same things from different perspectives. The more detailed your map is, the more freedom and flexibility you have.

- Do a reality check from time to time. Make sure that your map is up to date. When people stop looking at what's out there and rely on an old map, they mess up. Either they imagine limits and constraints where there are none or they continue to act as if something should work, and when it doesn't, they just do more of the same.

- Your future hasn't been written yet. Life is full of opportunities, and opportunities lie ahead, in the future. Don't let anyone, not even your own map, convince you of the contrary.

- It's not about who's right and who's wrong. It's not about what's true either. A good map is a map that gets you to see things from different perspectives and helps you feel as resourceful as possible about your situation.

- What people say they do or believe they do is often far removed from what they actually do.

- We have the mental tools and skills to get rid of the crap we don't want and replace it with what we do want.

- You can be whoever you choose to be.

- Change is the only constant in life. Are you going to choose the direction your life will take and the kind of person you will become or will you just sit back and wait for life to happen to you?

- People need someone who can 'speak their language', 'see things their way' or 'grasp their inner world'.

- If you want someone to access a certain state of mind, go there first. If you want a person to feel good, go into a wonderful state yourself.

- It's not your personal history that makes you who you are, it's your response to it.

- You can make every single thing you do magical, especially when you're with other people: just remember to go into the right state.

- The voices inside your head have volume controls. You can make them louder, you can make them softer, you can make them say what you want to – and in whatever tone of voice you choose.

- Get into the right state first. You can't be depressed and expect to help people be cheerful.

- If you go around grumpy, you will meet grumpy people or people will be grumpy around you. You reap what you sow.

- If you take problems too seriously, you just make them more real.

- States are contagious.

- If you go into the right state, you can do just about anything, but if you don't change your own internal state, then how can you expect anything to change?

- Shyness isn't a fixed personality trait. Shyness is just a state of mind.

- Building good feelings should be a part of how you do things every day.

- When you think about an unpleasant thing that has happened in your life, make sure it looks like a black-and-white Polaroid, then push it off into the distance and pretty soon it won't matter so much.

- People make the best choice they can at the time.

- If you want them to make better choices, help them expand their map of the world.

- Understand and respect others' maps.

- You have to take responsibility for your communication and if you're not getting the result you want, you need to change what you're doing.

- You affect others without even speaking to them. Your state affects their state (yoghurt knows yoghurt).

- Building rapport is a natural process.

- When two people get on really well, they tend to match each other's communication patterns at all levels, verbal and non-verbal.

- Matching means subtly and gradually adapting parts of your communication to that of the other person.

- When people communicate with you, they reveal how they are representing the world by the words that they use.

- Some of us prefer thinking in terms of visual images, others have a keen ear for sounds and words and some rely primarily on bodily sensations to make sense of the world. That doesn't mean we are that 'type' of person, but it does allow us to know how a person is thinking in that particular context.

- When you match the representational system someone is using, it makes them feel as though they are in rapport with you. When you mismatch it, they don't feel as good because they're not hearing what resonates with them.

- When we map reality, we delete, generalize and distort the information we receive from our senses. Then, when we describe that map with words, either to others or to ourselves, we do it again: we delete, generalize and distort the map.

- The more you drill down and identify the specific issue, the easier it is to help someone find a solution.

- The more you question a belief using the Meta Model, the more likely you are to sow seeds of doubt in the belief. That creates room for a person to change their belief to a more useful or resourceful one.

- When you find yourself in a difficult situation, the problem generally doesn't issue from the situation itself but from the way you think about it.

- Usually a person's problem isn't the most important problem. The biggest problem is that they spend so much time on it that if they do get rid of it, they just start filling their time up with new crap.

- In order to say no to something, your brain must first make an image of the thing you don't want and then negate it. The problem is that at this point you're already heading in the wrong direction.

- Disappointment requires adequate planning.

- If you begin to look at things as if they're difficult, they will be; if you begin to study what makes things impossible, you'll find out.

- People really need to learn to orient themselves towards a brighter future. And that begins by learning how to feel really good.

- The only time you ever lose is when you stop.

- If you are doing something and it's not working, there's got to be an easier way. And if what you're doing isn't working, you've got to do something else. And the first thing you've got to do is change your own internal state.

- You begin with your thoughts, then thoughts become actions, actions become habits, and habits become part of who you truly are.

Chapter 8

TECHNIQUES USED
IN THIS BOOK

Get Rid of Bad Memories

1. Think of something that recently happened to you and that
   still bothers you, something that you don't want to think of
   anymore. Focus on the visual representation of the memory
   – the image or movie that you see in your mind's eye.
2. Take that picture, make it smaller, move it off into the
   distance and drain the colour and brightness out of it.
3. If you hear the voices and sounds of the scene, make them
   fade away.
4. Make the picture so small you have to squint to see what's
   in there, and then make it even smaller.
5. When it's the size of a breadcrumb, you can just brush it
   away.

Trigger a Positive Feeling with the Skill of Anchoring

1. Imagine a movie screen right in front of you, so you can see your thoughts, and a lever connected to what you see on screen.
2. Go back in your mind to a really good experience. Feel the feelings you felt then.
3. Picture the image getting bigger and closer and more vivid as the feelings increase. As this happens, imagine a lever that says 'Fun' and slowly move it up. To make it feel even more real, make the gesture.
4. As you slide it up at the rate that fits the changes in your physiology and feelings, allow that exhilarating memory to get closer and closer and bigger and brighter.
5. Add colour to it. Make it shine. Look at the details.
6. Hear a voice in your head that says, 'Let the fun begin.'
7. Enjoy this wonderful sensation for an instant or two. Then pull the lever down to the initial position and let your body return to a more neutral state.
8. To verify that the anchoring was successful, stop for a moment and grab hold of that lever again, turning it up as you say to yourself, 'Let the fun begin.' You should go back to feeling as ecstatic as before.

Amplify Positive Feelings

1. Close your eyes and think about one of the best feelings you've ever had.
2. See what you saw and hear what you hear when you felt that good feeling.
3. As you do so, notice where this really amazing feeling comes from. Where in your body does it start? Where does it move to?
4. When you stop thinking about the feeling, where does it go?
5. Go back to that amazing feeling and let it come up. Just before it goes away, imagine pulling it out of your body and back to where it begins, so that it moves in a circle, and begin to spin it round and round, faster and faster.
6. Notice that as you spin it faster, the feeling gets stronger. How much pleasure your body is capable of?

Eliminate Negative Feelings

For this exercise you will need to tap into the amazing feeling you learned to amplify with the previous exercise.

1. Think about a part of your life where you feel stuck or blocked, something that gives you bad feelings and limits your behaviour.
2. Imagine watching it on a screen and taking hold of the brightness button. Then, in one quick move, turn it all the way bright, so you completely white it out. One moment you see it, and the next it's completely whited out.
3. Do it again. Imagine the thing that made you feel bad in this situation and white it out, really quickly.
4. Repeat the previous steps two or three times, until it comes naturally.
5. Take the amazing feeling you were working on before, and as you imagine the difficult situation in the future, again white out the negative image and spin this really good feeling around.
6. Hear an inner voice saying confidently, 'Never again!'
7. Focus on the good feeling spinning faster throughout your body – and notice what happens as your body fills with an incredible sense of well-being.
8. Shake your body in order to break the state and go back to a neutral state.

9. To verify that this new strategy works automatically, think about the negative situation and see how you feel about it. Can you imagine feeling bad?

Repeat this exercise until the new strategy works automatically.

The Power of Matching:
Non-verbal Communication

For this exercise you will need a partner.

Mismatching
1. Person A will talk about themselves.
2. Person B will listen, but mismatch person A's body language.
3. Person B will respond to something person A says, but at a different rate of speech and using a different representational system.
4. Meanwhile, person A will think about their experience and how it makes them feel about person B.

Matching
1. Person A will talk about themselves.
2. Person B will subtly match their body language, tone of voice, speed of speech and representational systems.
3. Person A will think about their experience and notice how it makes them feel about person B now.

Swap roles and ensure both of you get the chance to mismatch and match.

TECHNIQUES USED IN THIS BOOK

Meta-Model Questions

Use them to:

1. Specify information.
2. Clarify information.
3. Open up a person's model of the world.

The Questions
- How? What? When? Where? Who specifically?
- Who says? According to Whom?
- Everybody? Always? Never? Nobody? Nothing? All? No one?
- What do you mean by that?
- Compared to whom? Compared to what?
- How do you know?
- What stops you? What would happen if you could?
- What would happen if you did? What would happen if you didn't?

Building a Better Future

1. Allow your breathing to slow down and let yourself go effortlessly into a state of comfort.
2. Imagine time stretched out in front of you and behind you on a timeline. Imagine yourself drifting up above your timeline and looking down on your past, present and future.
3. As you look down at the past, you can see all those times when you had a bad experience. And as you look down at those experiences, you can realize that each of those experiences was a training ground for your future success.
4. Notice the useful information that emerges from each of those experiences. Let it float out above your timeline as a radiant glow. Take that light with you and leave the rest behind, in the past, where it belongs.
5. Next, think of a time when you were feeling on top of the world. Immerse yourself in that situation and let that fantastic sensation grow. Imagine it moving through your entire body.
6. Take this feeling, give it a colour of your choice and imagine spraying it through your past so that it covers every negative memory, every bad experience, soaking them in this really great feeling.
7. Imagine looking down and seeing how your past looks different now. Realize that you feel good about all those experiences. Whatever troubled you is now behind you and getting farther away by the second.

8. As you feel good about your past, imagine looking down at your future, and imagine the best kinds of feelings raining down on it, filling every future experience with the best states. See your future looking better than ever.

9. Float slowly back into your body, feeling full of excitement and anticipating the most amazing future, full of the most wonderful things – new people, new opportunities, new possibilities ... a world of possibilities.

A List of Submodalities

Here is a list of many of the submodalities (qualities) of the images, sounds and feelings of your thoughts.

Visual (Images, Movies)
- Associated (seeing through own eyes) or disassociated (seeing yourself in the image)
- Location: To the left, right, top, bottom
- Angle
- Number of pictures
- Size
- Distance
- Brightness
- Colour or monochrome (black and white)
- Framed (nature of frame?) or panoramic
- 2D or 3D
- Clear or fuzzy
- Shape: Convex, concave, specific shape
- Movement: Still, photo, slideshow, video, movie, looping
- Style: Picture, painting, poster, drawing, real life

Auditory (Sounds, Voices)
- Mono/stereo
- Tonality
- Qualities: Volume, pitch, tempo, rhythm, inflections, pauses, timbre

- Variations: Looping, fading in and out, moving location, moving direction
- Internal or external
- Voice: Whose voice? One or many
- Other background sounds?

Kinesthetic (Feelings)

- Vibration
- Pressure
- Steady or intermittent
- Intensity
- Weight
- Internal or external
- Location
- Shape
- Size
- Temperature
- Movement
- Texture

RESOURCES

Recommended Reading

Bandler, Richard, *Using Your Brain for a Change*, Real People Press, Durango, CO, 1985

_, *Magic in Action*, Meta Publications, Capitola, CA, 1985

_, *The Adventures of Anybody*, Meta Publications, Capitola, CA, 1993

_, *Time for a Change*, Meta Publications, Capitola, CA, 1993

_, *Get the Life You Want*, HarperElement, London, 2008

_, *Make Your Life Great*, HarperElement, London, 2010

Bandler, Richard, Delozier, Judith, and Grinder, John, *Patterns of the Hypnotic Techniques of Milton H. Erickson Volume 2*, Meta Publications, Capitola, CA, 1977

Bandler, Richard, and Grinder, John, *Frogs into Princes*, Real People Press, Capitola, CA, 1979

RESOURCES

_, *Patterns of the Hypnotic Techniques of Milton H. Erickson, Volume 1*, Meta Publications, Capitola, CA, 1975

_, *The Structure of Magic*, Meta Publications, Capitola, CA, 1975

_, *The Structure of Magic, Volume 2*, Meta Publications, Capitola, CA, 1975

_, *Trance-formations*, Real People Press, Durango, CO, 1980

Bandler, Richard, and Fitzpatrick, Owen, *Conversations with Richard Bandler*, Health Communications, Inc., Deerfield Beach, FL, 2009

Bandler, Richard, and La Valle, John, *Persuasion Engineering*, Meta Publications, Capitola, CA, 1996

Bandler, Richard, and McDonald, Will, *An Insider's Guide to Submodalities*, Meta Publications, Capitola, CA, 1989

Bandler, Richard, Roberti, Alessio, and Fitzpatrick, Owen, *Choose Freedom: Why Some People Live Happily and Others Don't.*

Fitzpatrick, Owen, *Not Enough Hours: The Secret to Making Every Second Count*, Poolbeg Press, Ltd, Dublin, 2009

Wilson, Robert Anton, *Prometheus Rising*, New Falcon Press, 1983

_, *Quantum Psychology*, New Falcon Press, 1990

DVD and CD Products

Bandler, Richard, *DHE*, CD, 2000

_, *The Art and Science of Nested Loops*, DVD, 2003

_, *Persuasion Engineering*, DVD, 2006

_, *Personal Enhancement Series*, CD, 2010
La Valle, John, *NLP Practitioner Set*, CD, 2009

These and many more DVDs and CDs, both hypnotic and from Richard's seminars, are available from www.nlpstore.com.

Bandler, Richard, *Adventures in Neuro Hypnotic
  Repatterning*, DVD set and PAL-version videos, 2002
_, *Thirty Years of NLP: How to Live a Happy Life*, DVD set,
  2003

These and other products by Richard Bandler are available from Matrix Essential Training Alliance, www.meta-nlp.co.uk; e-mail: enquiries@meta-nlp.co.uk; phone +44 (0)1749 871126; fax +44 (0)1749 870714

Fitzpatrick, Owen, *Love in Your Life*, Hypnosis CD, 2004
_, *Adventures in Charisma*, DVD set, 2008
_, *Performance Boost*, Hypnosis CD, 2011
_, *Confidence Boost*, Hypnosis CD, 2011

Available from www.nlp.ie

Websites

www.bandlervision.com
www.coach.tv
www.nlp.ie

RESOURCES

www.nlp.mobi
www.nlpcoach.com
www.NLPInstitutes.com
www.owenfitzpatrick.com
www.purenlp.com
www.richardbandler.com
www.theultimateintroductiontonlp.com

THE SOCIETY OF NEURO-LINGUISTIC PROGRAMMING

Richard Bandler Licensing Agreement

The Society of Neuro-Linguistic Programming is set up for the purpose of exerting quality control over those training programmes, services and materials claiming to represent the model of Neuro-Linguistic Programming (NLP). The seal below indicates Society Certification and is usually advertised by Society-approved trainers. When you purchase NLP products and seminars, ask to see this seal. This is your guarantee of quality.

It is common experience for many people when they are introduced to NLP and first begin to learn the technology, to be cautious and concerned with the possible uses and misuses.

As a protection for you and for those around you, the Society of NLP now requires participants to sign a licensing agreement which guarantees that those certified in this technology will use it with the highest integrity.

It is also a way to ensure that all the training you attend is of the highest quality and that your trainers are updated and current with the constant evolution of the field of Neuro-Linguistic Programming and Design Human Engineering, etc.

For a list of recommendations, go to:

- http://www.NLPInstitutes.com
- http://www.NLPTrainers.com
- http://www.NLPLinks.com

The Society of NLP
NLP™ Seminars Group International
PO Box 424
Hopatcong, NJ 07843
USA
Tel: (973) 770-3600
Website: www.purenlp.com

ABOUT THE AUTHORS

Dr Richard Bandler

Dr Richard Bandler is the co-founder of Neuro-Linguistic Programming and the creator of Design Human Engineering™ and Neuro Hypnotic Repatterning.™

For the last 40 years Dr Bandler has been one of the most important contributors to the field of personal change. A mathematician, philosopher, teacher, artist and composer, he has created a legacy of books, videos and audios that have changed therapy and education forever.

Hundreds of thousands of people, many of them therapists, have studied Dr Bandler's life's work at more than 600 institutes around the world.

A widely acclaimed keynote speaker and workshop leader, he is the author of more than a dozen books, including *Get the*

Life You Want, Make Your Life Great and *Using Your Brain for a Change*, and co-author of *Persuasion Engineering*,™ *Choose Freedom, The Secrets to Being Happy* and *Conversations with Richard Bandler*.

For more information on Richard Bandler's workshops and seminars visit www.richardbandler.com.

Alessio Roberti

Alessio Roberti is the International Director of Business Coaching for the Society of NLP, the largest NLP organization in the world. He has been studying Dr Richard Bandler's work for more than 20 years. He also attended Harvard Business School and Oxford Business School.

Alessio is a licensed Master Trainer of NLP and has trained more than 60,000 participants so far. He has coached presidents, CEOs, top executives and owners of some of the most important companies worldwide, in multiple industries.

He is the co-author, with Dr Bandler and Owen Fitzpatrick, of the book *Choose Freedom: Why Some People Live Happily and Others Don't*, which has been translated into seven languages. You can reach Alessio at www.coach.tv.

Owen Fitzpatrick

Owen Fitzpatrick is an international speaker and psychologist. He is the co-author of *Conversations with Richard Bandler* and *Choose Freedom* and the author of *Not Enough Hours: The Secret to Making Every Second Count.*

Owen also works with billionaires and Olympic athletes, helping them to perform at their very best. He is an authority in the area of charisma and motivation and he regularly delivers keynote speeches and corporate training on this topic.

As well as having a Master's in applied psychology, Owen has studied strategic negotiation at Harvard Business School and is a qualified psychotherapist and hypnotherapist. He is the co-founder of the Irish Institute of NLP. Owen also achieved the accolade of becoming the youngest ever licensed Master Trainer of NLP in the world, aged just 23.

Owen has travelled from Colombia to Japan and from Italy to Thailand and trained people in more than 20 countries worldwide in how to enhance their lives and improve their businesses.

You can find more information on Owen at www.owen-fitzpatrick.com or www.nlp.ie.